THE Skinny NUTRiBULLET

LEAN BODY YOGA PLAN

CookNation

THE SKINNY NUTRIBULLET LEAN BODY YOGA PLAN

DELICIOUS CALORIE COUNTED SMOOTHIES, JUICES AND GENTLE YOGA WORKOUTS FOR HEALTH & WELLBEING

ISBN 978-1-911219-36-1

A CIP catalogue record of this book is available from the British Library

DISCLAIMER

This book is designed to provide information on smoothies and juices that can be made in the NUTRiBULLET appliance only, results may differ if alternative devices are used.

A basic level of fitness is required to perform the workouts in this book. Any health concerns should be discussed with a health professional before embarking on any of the exercises detailed.

The NutriBullet™ is a registered trademark of Homeland Housewares, LLC. Bell & Mackenzie Publishing is not affiliated with the owner of the trademark and is not an authorized distributor of the trademark owner's products or services.
This publication has not been prepared, approved, or licensed by NutriBullet ™ or Homeland Housewares, LLC.

Some recipes may contain nuts or traces of nuts. Those suffering from any allergies associated with nuts should avoid any recipes containing nuts or nut based oils.
This information is provided and sold with the knowledge that the publisher and author do not offer any legal or other professional advice.
In the case of a need for any such expertise consult with the appropriate professional.
This book does not contain all information available on the subject, and other sources of recipes are available.

This book has not been created to be specific to any individual's or NUTRiBULLET's requirements.
Every effort has been made to make this book as accurate as possible. However, there may be typographical and or content errors. Therefore, this book should serve only as a general guide and not as the ultimate source of subject information.

This book contains information that might be dated and is intended only to educate and entertain.

The author and publisher shall have no liability or responsibility to any person or entity regarding any loss or damage incurred, or alleged to have incurred, directly or indirectly, by the information contained in this book.

CONTENTS

INTRODUCTION 7

NUTRIBLASTS UNDER 200 CALORIES 11

Super Green Banana Smoothie 12
Honey & Basil Juice 13
Ginger Apple Tonic Juice 14
Pineapple Pak Choi Smoothie 15
Strawberry Cashew Smoothie 16
Cauliflower Cleanser 17
Coconut Water Slushie 18
Papaya & Banana Smoothie 19
Double Berry Soya Smoothie 20
Blueberry Almond Milk 21
Carrot & Chia Nutri Juice 22
Rocket & Melon Milk Smoothie 23
Radish Vitamin C Smoothie 24
Mango & Almond Milk Smoothie 25
Sweet Pepper Apple Juice 26
Grapefruit & Goji Berries 27
Pumpkin Seed Apple Juice 28
Spirulina Green Smoothie 29
Ruby Coconut Water 30

NUTRIBLASTS UNDER 300 CALORIES 31

Pineapple Yoghurt Spiced Smoothie 32
Chia Peanut Butter Smoothie 33
Avocado, Banana Nut Smoothie 34
Mint & Grape Berry Juice 35
Mango Yoghurt Smoothie 36
Pumpkin Seed & Berry Smoothie 37
Banana & Date Almond Smoothie 38
Cashew Rich Milk Smoothie 39

Banana & Pumpkin Seed Smoothie 40
Avocado & Coconut Water Smoothie 41
Apple & Yoghurt Smoothie 42
Mixed Berry Almond Smoothie 43
Apple Turmeric Green Juice 44
Peanut Butter & Banana Smoothie 45
Broccoli & Chia Seed Smoothie 46
Kale & Coconut Milk Smoothie 47
Spring Time Smoothie 48
Double Nut Carrot Smoothie 49
Sweet Spinach Smoothie 50
Spicy Tomato Smoothie 51
Honey & Chia Seed Smoothie 52

NUTRIBLASTS UNDER 400 CALORIES **53**

Papaya & Banana Smoothie 54
Avocado Super Green Smoothie 55
Bright Herb Blast 56
Green Grape Good Juice 57
Grapefruit & Pineapple Sweet Juice 58
Peach Cashew Smoothie 59
Carrot & Kale Cleanser 60
Spring Goji Berry Smoothie 61
Chia & Soya Pineapple Smoothie 62
Walnut Blueberry Smoothie 63
Cherry Green Smoothie 64
Pineapple Protein Shake 65
Fresh Almond & Pear Smoothie 66
Oat & Chia Seed Morning Blaster 67
Beetroot & Orange Protein Smoothie 68
Green Green Soya Milk Smoothie 69
Kale & Coconut Milk Smoothie 70
Banana & Hemp Seed Smoothie 71
Vanilla & Date Coconut Smoothie 72
Almond Butter Spinach Smoothie 73

Hemp & Almond Milk Smoothie 74

YOGA WORKOUTS **75**

Morning Yoga 76

Tummy Toning Yoga 84

Restful Sleep Yoga 90

OTHER COOKNATION TITLES **95**

INTRODUCTION

Our nutritious smoothies and yoga workouts are a healthy combination which will set you on the path to enhanced well being.

If you are reading this you will likely already have purchased a NUTRiBULLET or perhaps are considering buying one. A smart choice! The NUTRiBULLET is unquestionably one of the highest performing smoothie creators on the market. Its clean lines and compact design look great in any kitchen. It's simple to use, easy to clean and the results are amazing.

You may have watched or read some of the NUTRiBULLET marketing videos and literature which make claims of using the power of the NUTRiBULLET to help you lose weight, boost your immune system and fight a number of ailments and diseases. Of course the 'healing' power comes from the foods we use to make our smoothies but the real difference with the NUTRiBULLET is that it EXTRACTS all the goodness of the ingredients. Unlike many juicers and blenders, which leave behind valuable fibre, the NUTRiBULLET pulverises the food, breaking down their cell walls and unlocking the valuable nutrients so your body can absorb and use them.

You may have made your own smoothies in the past using a blender – you'll know even with a powerful device that there are often indigestible pieces of food left in your glass – not so with the NUTRiBULLET which uses 600 watts to breakdown every part of the food. The manufacturer calls it 'cyclonic action' running at 10,000 revolutions per minute but whatever the marketing jargon, the results speak for themselves.

The NUTRiBULLET is not a blender and not a juicer. It is a nutrient extractor, getting the very best from every ingredient you put in and delivering a nutrient packed smoothie called a 'Nutriblast'. Using the power of the NUTRiBULLET is an incredibly fast and efficient way of giving our bodies the goodness they need. Making the most of anti-oxidants to protect your cells, omega 3 fatty acids to help your joints, fibre to aid digestion and protein to build and repair muscles.

Just one nutrient packed Nutriblast a day can make a difference to the way you feel and it only takes seconds to make!

All our recipes make use of the tall cup of the NUTRiBULLET and the extractor blade. Feel free to experiment. Mixing your ingredients is fun and will help your create wonderful new combinations too. As a basic formula, work on 50% leafy greens 50% fruit, ¼ cup of seeds/nuts and water.

There has never been a better time to introduce health-boosting, weight reducing, well-being smoothies to your life. With a spiralling obesity epidemic in the western world which in turn is linked to a growing list of debilitating diseases and ailments including diabetes, high blood pressure, heart disease, high cholesterol, infertility, skin conditions and more, the future for many of us can look bleak. Combine this with the super-fast pace of modern life and we can be left feeling fatigued and lethargic, worsened by daily consumption of unhealthy foods.

The good news is that you have taken a positive step to improve your life. The power of the NUTRiBULLET, our delicious calorie counted smoothies and yoga workouts are a healthy combination which will set you on the path to enhanced well being. You should however not rely solely on our recipes as your daily nutritional intake. Physical and indeed everyday activities require energy to perform so we recommend a balanced diet of carbohydrates, protein and fat. Using a fitness tracker such as MyFitnessPal will help you achieve your daily nutritional needs.

YOGA

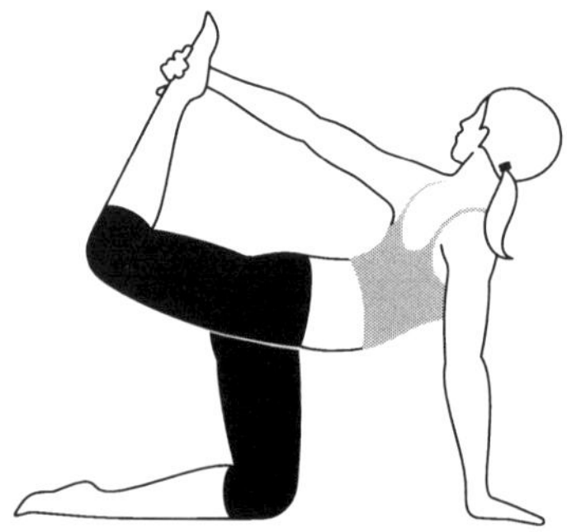

Yoga is an ancient form of exercise that focuses on strength, flexibility and breathing. Originating in India more than 5,000 years ago, yoga is practiced to boost physical & mental wellbeing and has been adopted by cultures around the world.

It is a safe and effective way to increase physical activity, especially strength, flexibility and balance. Yoga is thought to have many healing properties and is beneficial for people with high blood pressure, heart disease, aches and pains, depression and stress.

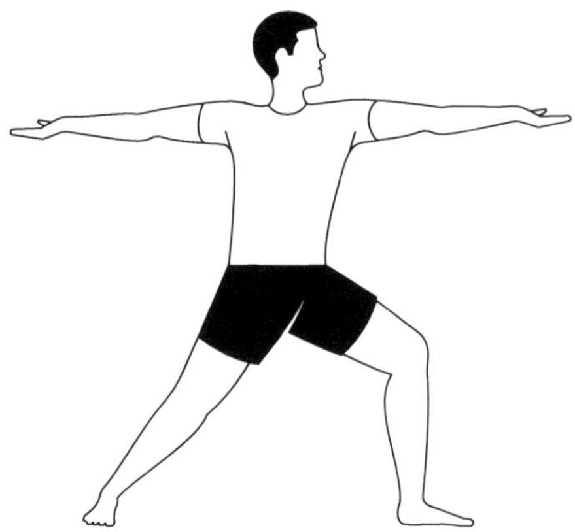

There are a number of different types of yoga which are generally practiced including Hatha, Vinyasa & Iyengar to name just three. The routines which have been developed for this book are not confined to one type of yoga and will give you a basic introduction to this wonderful form of exercise.

You will find three yoga workouts in this book. The first 2 routines will take around 15 minutes to complete. The third is a 30 minute relaxation session. Incorporating a yoga routine into your daily life will benefit you both physically and mentally. All you need to get started is a mat, a block and pillows for support (for the relaxation routine at the end). That said there is not need to run out and buy any equipment at all. You can do any of these routines comfortably on a rug or carpet and the yoga block can be substituted for a small strong shoe sized box.

Yoga will, in time, help you 'still' your mind. When you are doing the routines try to empty your brain of any thoughts. That is not as easy as it sounds, but have patience with yourself. If you try to anchor your thoughts around your breathing you will learn to calm your mind and move towards a stillness which will benefit your well being.

Enjoy your yoga journey.

YOGA TIPS

- A few things to remember:
- Yoga should never be approached as a competitive sport. It is a personal journey. Always listen to your body and never push yourself too hard. Concentrating on breathing is an extremely important part of yoga practice and you will learnt to use the rhythm of your breathing to help you move through the poses.
- Always move into poses on a breath exhalation and make sure you move slowly and methodically.

NUTRIBULLET TIPS

To help make your Nutriblast fuss-free, follow these quick tips.

- Prepare your shopping list. Take some time to select which Nutriblasts you want to prepare in advance. As with all food shopping, make a note of all the ingredients and quantities you need. Depending on the ingredients it's best not to shop too far in advance to ensure you are getting the freshest produce available. We recommend buying organic produce whenever you can if your budget allows. Organic produce can give a better yield and flavour to your Nutriblast. Remember almost all fruit is fine to freeze too.
- Wash your fruit and veg before juicing. This needn't take up much time but all produce should be washed clean of any traces of bacteria, pesticides and insects.
- To save time prepare produce the night before for early morning Nutriblasts.
- Cut up any produce that may not fit into the tall cup, but only do this just before making your smoothie to keep it as fresh as possible.
- Wash your Nutriblast parts immediately after juicing. As tempting as it may be to leave it till a little later you'll be glad you took the few minutes to rinse and wash before any residue has hardened.
- Substitute where you need to. If you can't source a particular ingredient, try another instead. More often than not you will find the use of a different fruit or veg makes a really interesting and delicious alternative. In our recipes we offer some advice on alternatives but have the confidence to make your own too!
- Some Nutriblasts are sweeter than others and it's a fact that some of the leafy green drinks can take a little getting used to. Try drinking these with a straw, you'll find them easier to drink and enjoy.

IMPORTANT – WHAT NOT TO USE IN YOUR NUTRIBLASTS

The manufacturers of NUTRiBULLET are very clear on the following warning. While the joy of making Nutriblasts is using whole fruit and vegetables there are a few seeds and pits which should be removed. The following contain chemicals which can release cyanide into the body when ingested so do not use any of the following in your Nutriblasts:

- **Apple Seeds**
- **Cherry Pits**
- **Peach pits**
- **Apricot Pits**
- **Plum Pits**

CLEANING

- Cleaning the NUTRiBULLET is thankfully very easy. The manufacturer gives clear guidelines on how best to do this but here's a recap:
- Make sure the NUTRiBULLET is unplugged before disassembling or cleaning.
- Set aside the power base and blade holders as these should not be used in a dishwasher.
- Use hot soapy water to clean the blades but do not immerse in boiling water as this can warp the plastic.
- Use a damp cloth to clean the power base.
- All cups and lids can be placed in a dishwasher.
- For stubborn marks inside the cup, fill the cup 2/3 full of warm soapy water and screw on the milling blade. Attach to the power base and run for 20-30 seconds.

WARNING:

Do not put your hands or any utensils near the moving blade. Always ensure the NUTRiBULLET is unplugged when assembling/disassembling or cleaning.

ABOUT CookNation

CookNation is the leading publisher of innovative and practical recipe books for the modern, health conscious cook.

CookNation titles bring together delicious, easy and practical recipes with their unique approach - easy and delicious, no-nonsense recipes - making cooking for diets and healthy eating fast, simple and fun.

With a range of #1 best-selling titles - from the innovative 'Skinny' calorie-counted series, to the 5:2 Diet Recipes collection - CookNation recipe books prove that 'Diet' can still mean 'Delicious'!

THE Skinny NUTRiBULLET LEAN BODY YOGA PLAN

NUTRIBLASTS UNDER 200 CALORIES

SERVES 1

SUPER GREEN BANANA SMOOTHIE

170 calories

Ingredients

- 50g/2oz kale
- 25g/1oz spinach
- ¼ cucumber
- 1 banana
- 2 tsp flax seeds
- Water

Method

1 Rinse the ingredients well.

2 Cut any thick green stalks off the spinach and kale.

3 Nip the ends off the cucumber but don't bother peeling.

4 Add the greens, cucumber, banana & flax seeds to the NUTRiBULLET tall cup. Make sure the ingredients do not go past the MAX line on your machine.

5 Add water, again being careful not to exceed the MAX line.

6 Twist on the NUTRiBULLET blade and blend until smooth.

CHEF'S NOTE

This smoothie is bursting with green goodness. Add a little apple is you need extra natural sweetness.

SERVES 1

HONEY & BASIL JUICE

165 calories

Ingredients

- 3 tbsp fresh basil leaves
- 50g/2oz spinach
- 1 apple
- 2 tsp honey
- Water

Method

1. Rinse the ingredients well.
2. Cut any thick stalks off the spinach. Core the apple.
3. Add the basil, spinach, apple & honey to the NUTRiBULLET tall cup. Make sure the ingredients do not go past the MAX line on your machine.
4. Add water, again being careful not to exceed the MAX line.
5. Twist on the NUTRiBULLET blade and blend until smooth.

CHEF'S NOTE

A little fresh mint is also good added to this simple sweet juice.

SERVES 1

GINGER APPLE TONIC JUICE

160 calories

Ingredients

- 50g/2oz spinach
- 125g/4oz carrot
- 2cm/1 inch fresh peeled ginger root
- 1 apple
- Water

Method

1 Rinse the ingredients well.

2 Cut any thick green stalks off the spinach.

3 Core the apple. Top & tail the carrots, no need to peel.

4 Add the fruit, vegetables & ginger to the NUTRiBULLET tall cup. Make sure the ingredients do not go past the MAX line on your machine.

5 Add water, again being careful not to exceed the MAX line.

6 Twist on the NUTRiBULLET blade and blend until smooth.

CHEF'S NOTE

Apple and ginger work together to make a vibrant antioxidant juice combo.

SERVES 1

PINEAPPLE PAK CHOI SMOOTHIE

195 calories

Ingredients

NUTRIENT DENSE

- 75g/3oz pak choi/bok choi
- 150g/5oz fresh pineapple
- 1 banana
- Water

Method

1. Rinse the ingredients well.
2. Peel the banana. Cut any thick woody ends off the pak choi.
3. Add the fruit & vegetables to the NUTRiBULLET tall cup. Make sure the ingredients do not go past the MAX line on your machine.
4. Add water, again being careful not to exceed the MAX line.
5. Twist on the NUTRiBULLET blade and blend until smooth.

CHEF'S NOTE

Use tinned pineapple if you don't have fresh pineapple.

STRAWBERRY CASHEW SMOOTHIE

SERVES 1

198 calories

Ingredients

- 50g/2oz spinach
- 150g/5oz strawberries
- 5 cashew nuts
- 250ml/1 cup unsweetened almond milk
- Water

Method

1 Rinse the ingredients well.

2 Cut any thick green stalks off the spinach and remove the green tops from the strawberries.

3 Add the spinach, fruit & nuts to the NUTRiBULLET tall cup. Make sure the ingredients do not go past the MAX line on your machine.

4 Add water, again being careful not to exceed the MAX line.

5 Twist on the NUTRiBULLET blade and blend until smooth.

CHEF'S NOTE

Cashew nuts contain vitamins E, K, and B6, along with copper, phosphorus, zinc, magnesium & iron.

CAULIFLOWER CLEANSER

SERVES 1

175 calories

Ingredients

- 125g/4oz cauliflower florets
- 50g/2oz watercress
- 250ml/1 cup unsweetened almond milk
- 2 tsp honey
- Water

Method

1 Rinse the ingredients well.

2 Add the cauliflower, watercress, honey & almond milk to the NUTRiBULLET tall cup. Make sure the ingredients do not go past the MAX line on your machine.

3 Add water, again being careful not to exceed the MAX line.

4 Twist on the NUTRiBULLET blade and blend until smooth.

CHEF'S NOTE

Cauliflower is a great source of Vitamin C.

SERVES 1

COCONUT WATER SLUSHIE

170 calories

Ingredients

- 75g/3oz spinach
- 1 banana
- 250ml/1 cup coconut water
- Handful of ice cubes

NUTRIENT RICH

Method

1 Rinse the spinach well and cut off any thick stalks.

2 Peel the banana.

3 Add the spinach, banana & coconut water to the NUTRiBULLET tall cup along with ice cubes. Make sure the ingredients do not go past the MAX line on your machine.

4 Twist on the NUTRiBULLET blade and blend until smooth.

CHEF'S NOTE

Always use unsweetened 100% coconut water.

SERVES 1

PAPAYA & BANANA SMOOTHIE

160 calories

Ingredients

AIDS DIGESTION

- 25g/1oz spinach
- 1 papaya
- 1 banana
- Water

Method

1 Rinse the ingredients well.

2 Peel the banana.

3 Add all the ingredients to the NUTRiBULLET tall cup. Make sure the contents do not go past the MAX line on your machine.

4 Add water, again being careful not to exceed the MAX line.

5 Twist on the NUTRiBULLET blade and blend until smooth.

CHEF'S NOTE

Papaya is high in fibre which helps promote a healthy digestive tract.

SERVES 1

DOUBLE BERRY SOYA SMOOTHIE

165 calories

Ingredients

- 50g/2oz raspberries
- 50g/2oz strawberries
- 250ml/1 cup soya milk
- Water

VITAMIN C +

Method

1 Rinse the ingredients well. Nip any green tops off the strawberries.

2 Add the fruit & milk to the NUTRiBULLET tall cup. Make sure the ingredients do not go past the MAX line on your machine.

3 Add water, again being careful not to exceed the MAX line.

4 Twist on the NUTRiBULLET blade and blend until smooth.

CHEF'S NOTE

Adjust the quantity of water to get the consistency you prefer.

BLUEBERRY ALMOND MILK

SERVES 1

175 calories

Ingredients

- 50g/3oz tenderstem broccoli/broccolini
- 75g/3oz blueberries
- 1 tsp honey
- 250ml/1 cup unsweetened almond milk
- Water

Method

1 Rinse the ingredients well.

2 Cut any thick woody ends off the broccoli.

3 Add the fruit, vegetables, honey and milk to the NUTRiBULLET tall cup. Make sure the ingredients do not go past the MAX line on your machine.

4 Add water, again being careful not to exceed the MAX line.

5 Twist on the NUTRiBULLET blade and blend until smooth.

CHEF'S NOTE

Tenderstem broccoli is an excellent source of Vitamins K & C.

SERVES 1

CARROT & CHIA NUTRI JUICE

190 calories

Ingredients

- 200g/7oz carrots
- 1 apple
- 1 tbsp chia seeds
- Water

OMEGA 3+

Method

1 Rinse the ingredients well.

2 Top & tail the carrots, no need to peel. Core the apple.

3 Add the carrots, apple & chia seeds to the NUTRiBULLET tall cup. Make sure the ingredients do not go past the MAX line on your machine.

4 Add water, again being careful not to exceed the MAX line.

5 Twist on the NUTRiBULLET blade and blend until smooth.

CHEF'S NOTE

Chia seeds are prized for their high protein and essential fatty acid content.

SERVES 1

ROCKET & MELON MILK SMOOTHIE

155 calories

Ingredients

POTASSIUM RICH

- 25g/1oz rocket
- 200g/7oz melon flesh
- 250ml/1 cup soya milk
- Water

Method

1 Rinse the ingredients well.

2 Add the melon, rocket & milk to the NUTRiBULLET tall cup. Make sure the ingredients do not go past the MAX line on your machine.

3 Add a little water if needed to take it up to the MAX line.

4 Twist on the NUTRiBULLET blade and blend until smooth.

CHEF'S NOTE

Rocket has a unique peppery taste which adds an unusual dimension to this smoothie.

RADISH VITAMIN C SMOOTHIE

SERVES 1

193 calories

Ingredients

- 50g/2oz spinach
- 1 orange
- 75g/3oz radishes
- 250ml/1 cup unsweetened almond milk
- Water

Method

1 Rinse the ingredients well.

2 Cut any thick green stalks off the spinach.

3 Peel and de-seed the orange.

4 Nip the tops of the radishes.

5 Add the fruit, vegetables & almond milk to the NUTRiBULLET tall cup. Make sure the ingredients do not go past the MAX line on your machine.

6 Add a little water if needed to take it up to the MAX line.

7 Twist on the NUTRiBULLET blade and blend until smooth.

CHEF'S NOTE

Radishes are good sources and folate, fibre and potassium.

SERVES 1

MANGO & ALMOND MILK SMOOTHIE

190 calories

Ingredients

GOOD ENZYMES

- 50g/2oz spinach
- 125g/4oz mango
- 250ml/1 cup unsweetened almond milk
- Water

Method

1 Rinse the ingredients well.

2 Cut any thick green stalks off the spinach.

3 Peel and stone the mango.

4 Add the mango, spinach & almond milk to the NUTRiBULLET tall cup. Make sure the ingredients do not go past the MAX line on your machine.

5 Add a little water if needed to take it up to the MAX line.

6 Twist on the NUTRiBULLET blade and blend until smooth.

CHEF'S NOTE

Almond milk is low in fat, high in energy, proteins, lipids and fibre.

SERVES 1

SWEET PEPPER APPLE JUICE

190 calories

Ingredients

- 50g/2oz spinach
- 1 yellow pepper
- 1 apple
- 50g/2oz carrots
- Water

Method

1 Rinse the ingredients well.

2 Remove any thick stalks from the spinach.

3 De-seed and core the yellow pepper & apple. Nip the ends of the carrots and peel.

4 Add the fruit & vegetables to the NUTRiBULLET tall cup. Make sure the ingredients do not go past the MAX line on your machine.

5 Add water, again being careful not to exceed the MAX line.

6 Twist on the NUTRiBULLET blade and blend until smooth.

CHEF'S NOTE

Peppers are a surprisingly good source of Vitamin C.

SERVES 1

GRAPEFRUIT & GOJI BERRIES

148 calories

Ingredients

- 1 grapefruit
- 2 sprigs fresh mint
- 2 tbsp goji berries
- 1 tsp honey
- Ice

Method

1. Peel and de-seed the grapefruit. Rinse the mint.
2. Add everything to the NUTRiBULLET tall cup, finishing with ice. Make sure the ingredients do not go past the MAX line on your machine.
3. Twist on the NUTRiBULLET blade and blend until smooth.

CHEF'S NOTE

Grapefruit is mineral and vitamin rich.

SERVES 1

PUMPKIN SEED APPLE JUICE

164 calories

Ingredients

- 75g/3oz spinach
- 1 apple
- 2 tsp pumpkin seeds
- 1 tsp lemon juice
- Water

Method

1. Rinse the spinach and apple. Core the apple, don't peel.
2. Add the ingredients to the NUTRiBULLET tall cup, finishing with water to taste. Make sure not to pass the MAX line on your machine.
3. Twist on the NUTRiBULLET blade and blend until smooth.

CHEF'S NOTE

Try using a pear instead of an apple.

SERVES 1

SPIRULINA GREEN SMOOTHIE

175
calories

Ingredients

- 50g/2oz spinach
- 2 celery stalks
- ½ tsp spirulina
- 120ml/½ cup light coconut milk
- Water

Method

1. Rinse the spinach and the celery. Chop the celery and remove any thick stems from the spinach. Add to the NUTRiBULLET tall cup.
2. Add the spirulina and coconut milk. Fill with water to the MAX line on your machine.
3. Twist on the NUTRiBULLET blade and blend until smooth.

CHEF'S NOTE

Spirulina is a great source of nutrients including vitamins B, C, D, A and E.

SERVES 1

RUBY COCONUT WATER

190 calories

Ingredients

- ½ fresh beetroot
- 1 apple
- 75g/3oz strawberries
- 250ml/1 cup coconut water
- Water

ANTIOXIDANTS

Method

1 Rinse the strawberries and nip off any green tops.

2 Core the apple. Peel the beetroot and add to the NUTRiBULLET tall cup along with the strawberries.

3 Pour in the coconut water. Make sure the ingredients do not go past the MAX line on your machine.

4 Add a little water if needed to take it up to the MAX line.

5 Twist on the NUTRiBULLET blade and blend until smooth.

CHEF'S NOTE

Raw or cooked beetroot will work well for this juice (but not pickled).

THE Skinny NUTRiBULLET LEAN BODY YOGA PLAN

NUTRIBLASTS UNDER 300 CALORIES

SERVES 1

PINEAPPLE YOGHURT SPICED SMOOTHIE

275 calories

Ingredients

- 200g/7oz pineapple
- 2 tbsp Greek yoghurt
- 250ml/1 cup unsweetened almond milk
- 2cm/1 inch peeled fresh ginger root
- Pinch ground cinnamon
- Handful of ice
- Water

Method

1. Add the pineapple, yoghurt, milk, ginger, cinnamon and & ice to the NUTRiBULLET tall cup. Make sure the ingredients do not go past the MAX line on your machine.
2. Add a little water if needed to take it up to the MAX line.
3. Twist on the NUTRiBULLET blade and blend until smooth.

CHEF'S NOTE

Ginger and cinnamon are believed to help aid digestion.

SERVES 1

CHIA PEANUT BUTTER SMOOTHIE

260 calories

Ingredients

- 1 tbsp reduced fat peanut butter
- 250ml/1 cup unsweetened almond milk
- 1 tbsp oats
- 1 tbsp chia seeds
- Water

Method

1 Add the peanut butter, milk, oats & chia seeds to the NUTRiBULLET tall cup. Make sure the ingredients do not go past the MAX line on your machine.

2 Add a little water if needed to take it up to the MAX line.

3 Twist on the NUTRiBULLET blade and blend until smooth.

CHEF'S NOTE

Chia seeds and oats will release energy in your body slowly throughout the day.

SERVES 1

AVOCADO, BANANA NUT SMOOTHIE

295 calories

Ingredients

- ¼ ripe avocado
- 1 banana
- 6 walnut halves
- 250ml/1 cup unsweetened almond milk
- Water

Method

1 Rinse the ingredients well.

2 Peel & stone the avocado. Peel the banana.

3 Add the avocado, banana, walnuts & milk to the NUTRiBULLET tall cup. Make sure the ingredients do not go past the MAX line on your machine.

4 Add water, again being careful not to exceed the MAX line.

5 Twist on the NUTRiBULLET blade and blend until smooth.

CHEF'S NOTE

Rich and nutty this simple smoothie packs an energy punch.

SERVES 1

MINT & GRAPE BERRY JUICE

255 calories

Ingredients

- 150g/5oz raspberries
- 150g/5oz seedless green grapes
- 1 banana
- 2 fresh mint leaves
- Water

Method

1 Rinse the ingredients well.

2 Peel the banana.

3 Add the fruit and mint to the NUTRiBULLET tall cup. Make sure the ingredients do not go past the MAX line on your machine.

4 Add water, again being careful not to exceed the MAX line.

5 Twist on the NUTRiBULLET blade and blend until smooth.

CHEF'S NOTE

A handful of spinach or kale adds a little green goodness to this sweet fruit juice.

SERVES 1

MANGO YOGHURT SMOOTHIE

295 calories

Ingredients

- 200g/7oz mango
- 2 tbsp Greek yoghurt
- 180ml/¾ cup semi skimmed milk
- 1 tsp honey
- Water

Method

1 Peel and stone the mango.

2 Add the mango, yoghurt, milk & honey to the NUTRiBULLET tall cup. Make sure the ingredients do not go past the MAX line on your machine.

3 Add water, again being careful not to exceed the MAX line.

4 Twist on the NUTRiBULLET blade and blend until smooth.

CHEF'S NOTE

Try adding a handful of ice cubes too.

SERVES 1

PUMPKIN SEED & BERRY SMOOTHIE

293 calories

Ingredients

- 50g/2oz spinach
- 150g/5oz strawberries
- 1 banana
- 250ml/1 cup unsweetened almond milk
- 1 tbsp pumpkin seeds
- Water

Method

1 Rinse the ingredients well.

2 Remove any green tops from the strawberries.

3 Peel the banana.

4 Add the spinach, fruit, soya milk & pumpkin seeds to the NUTRiBULLET tall cup. Make sure the ingredients do not go past the MAX line on your machine.

5 Add a little water if needed to take it up to the MAX line.

6 Twist on the NUTRiBULLET blade and blend until smooth.

CHEF'S NOTE

For an additional protein blast add a scoop of protein powder.

SERVES 1

BANANA & DATE ALMOND SMOOTHIE

285 calories

Ingredients

- 1 banana
- 4 pitted dates
- 250ml/1 cup unsweetened almond milk
- 1 tsp lime juice
- 1 pinch ground cinnamon
- Water

Method

1 Peel the banana.

2 Add the banana, dates, milk, lime juice & cinnamon to the NUTRiBULLET tall cup. Make sure the ingredients do not go past the MAX line on your machine.

3 Add a little water if needed to take it up to the MAX line.

4 Twist on the NUTRiBULLET blade and blend until smooth.

CHEF'S NOTE

Use dried unsweetened dates and ensure all the stones are removed.

SERVES 1

CASHEW RICH MILK SMOOTHIE

270 calories

Ingredients

- 1 banana
- 250ml/1 cup unsweetened almond milk
- Pinch ground cinnamon
- 10 cashew nuts
- Water

Method

1 Peel the banana.

2 Add the banana, cashews, cinnamon & almond milk to the NUTRiBULLET tall cup. Make sure the ingredients do not go past the MAX line on your machine.

3 Add a little water if needed to take it up to the MAX line.

4 Twist on the NUTRiBULLET blade and blend until smooth.

CHEF'S NOTE

Add more cashew nuts if you wish.

SERVES 1

BANANA & PUMPKIN SEED SMOOTHIE

270 calories

Ingredients

- 50g/2oz spinach
- 1 banana
- 250ml/1 cup soya milk
- 1 tbsp pumpkin seeds
- Water

Method

1. Rinse the ingredients well.
2. Cut any thick green stalks off the spinach.
3. Peel the banana.
4. Add the spinach, bananas, milk & pumpkin seeds to the NUTRiBULLET tall cup. Make sure the ingredients do not go past the MAX line on your machine.
5. Add a little water if needed to take it up to the MAX line.
6. Twist on the NUTRiBULLET blade and blend until smooth.

CHEF'S NOTE

Soya milk is naturally high in essential fatty acids, proteins, fibre, vitamins and minerals.

SERVES 1

AVOCADO & COCONUT WATER SMOOTHIE

299 calories

Ingredients

- 50g/2oz spinach
- ½ avocado
- 1 apple
- 250ml/1 cup coconut water
- Water

Method

1 Rinse the ingredients well.

2 Remove any thick stalks from the spinach.

3 Peel & stone the avocado. Core the apple.

4 Add the fruit, vegetables & coconut water to the NUTRiBULLET tall cup. Make sure the ingredients do not go past the MAX line on your machine.

5 Add a little water if needed to take it up to the MAX line.

6 Twist on the NUTRiBULLET blade and blend until smooth.

CHEF'S NOTE

Avocado and spinach combine for a vitamin rich smoothie.

SERVES 1

APPLE & YOGHURT SMOOTHIE

206 calories

Ingredients

- 1 apple
- 4 tbsp Greek yoghurt
- 1 tsp lime juice
- 1 tsp chia seeds
- Water

Method

1. Rinse and core the apple.
2. Add the apple, yoghurt, lime juice & chia seeds to the NUTRiBULLET tall cup. Make sure the ingredients do not go past the MAX line on your machine.
3. Add water, again being careful not to exceed the MAX line.
4. Twist on the NUTRiBULLET blade and blend until smooth.

CHEF'S NOTE

Adjust the lime to suit your own taste in this creamy smoothie.

SERVES 1

MIXED BERRY ALMOND SMOOTHIE

285 calories

Ingredients

- 25g/1oz spinach
- 150g/5oz mixed berries
- 1 banana
- 250ml/1 cup unsweetened almond milk
- Water

Method

1 Rinse the ingredients well.

2 Peel the banana.

3 Add the spinach, fruit & almond milk to the NUTRiBULLET tall cup. Make sure the ingredients do not go past the MAX line on your machine.

4 Add a little water if needed to take it up to the MAX line.

5 Twist on the NUTRiBULLET blade and blend until smooth.

CHEF'S NOTE

Try this recipe using cranberries instead of mixed berries.

SERVES 1

APPLE TURMERIC GREEN JUICE

240 calories

Ingredients

- 1 apple
- 200g/7oz carrots
- ½ tsp ground turmeric
- 250ml/1 cup coconut water
- Ice cubes

Method

1. Rinse the ingredients well.
2. Core the apple.
3. Nip the ends off the carrots, don't bother peeling.
4. Add the fruit, vegetables, turmeric & coconut water to the NUTRiBULLET tall cup. Make sure the ingredients do not go past the MAX line on your machine.
5. Add ice cubes, again being careful not to exceed the MAX line.
6. Twist on the NUTRiBULLET blade and blend until smooth.

CHEF'S NOTE

Turmeric is a natural anti-inflammatory which has been used in Chinese medicine throughout the ages.

SERVES 1

PEANUT BUTTER & BANANA SMOOTHIE

265 calories

Ingredients

- 1 banana
- 1 tbsp peanut butter
- 120ml/½ cup semi skimmed milk
- Handful of ice cubes
- Water

Method

1 Peel the banana.

2 Add the banana, peanut butter and ice cubes to the NUTRiBULLET tall cup. Make sure the ingredients do not go past the MAX line on your machine.

3 Add water, again being careful not to exceed the MAX line.

4 Twist on the NUTRiBULLET blade and blend until smooth.

CHEF'S NOTE

Soya milk also works well in this protein rich banana smoothie.

SERVES 1

BROCCOLI & CHIA SEED SMOOTHIE

297 calories

Ingredients

- 125g/4oz tenderstem broccoli/broccolini
- 1 apple
- 1 banana
- 1 tbsp chia seeds
- Water

Method

1. Rinse the ingredients well.
2. Core the apple and peel the banana.
3. Add the broccoli, apple, banana & chia seeds to the NUTRiBULLET tall cup. Make sure the ingredients do not go past the MAX line on your machine.
4. Add water, again being careful not to exceed the MAX line.
5. Twist on the NUTRiBULLET blade and blend until smooth.

CHEF'S NOTE

Chia seeds are nutrient dense and pack a serious energy punch.

SERVES 1

KALE & COCONUT MILK SMOOTHIE

260 calories

Ingredients

FIBRE RICH

- 50g/2oz kale
- 180ml/¾ cup light coconut milk
- ½ banana
- Water

Method

1 Rinse the ingredients well.

2 Remove any thick stalks from the kale.

3 Peel the banana.

4 Add the kale, banana & coconut milk to the NUTRiBULLET tall cup. Make sure the ingredients do not go past the MAX line on your machine.

5 Add a little water if needed to take it up to the MAX line.

6 Twist on the NUTRiBULLET blade and blend until smooth.

CHEF'S NOTE

Use low fat coconut milk, it's not as creamy as the full fat version but is much lower in calories.

SERVES 1

SPRING TIME SMOOTHIE

298 calories

Ingredients

- 75g/3oz shredded spring cabbage greens
- 1 banana
- 1 apple
- 120ml/½ cup soya milk
- Water

Method

1. Rinse the ingredients well.
2. Core the apple and peel the banana.
3. Add the greens, fruit & milk to the NUTRiBULLET tall cup. Make sure the ingredients do not go past the MAX line on your machine.
4. Add water, again being careful not to exceed the MAX line.
5. Twist on the NUTRiBULLET blade and blend until smooth.

CHEF'S NOTE

Spring greens are the first cabbages of the year. They have loose heads without the tough core of other cabbages.

SERVES 1

DOUBLE NUT CARROT SMOOTHIE

240 calories

Ingredients

- 150g/5oz carrots
- 125g/4oz strawberries
- 250ml/1 cup unsweetened almond milk
- 1 tbsp almonds
- Water

Method

1 Rinse the ingredients well.

2 Top & tail the carrots, no need to peel. Nip any green tops off the strawberries.

3 Add the carrots, strawberries, almond milk & ground almonds to the NUTRiBULLET tall cup. Make sure the ingredients do not go past the MAX line on your machine.

4 Add a little water if needed to take it up to the MAX line.

5 Twist on the NUTRiBULLET blade and blend until smooth.

CHEF'S NOTE

Almonds are a good source of Vitamin E.

SERVES 1

SWEET SPINACH SMOOTHIE

240 calories

Ingredients

- 50g/2oz spinach
- 250ml/1 cup coconut water
- 200g/7oz pineapple
- Water

AIDS DIGESTION

Method

1 Rinse the spinach well.

2 Peel the pineapple and cut into chunks.

3 Add all the ingredients to the NUTRiBULLET tall cup. Make sure they do not go past the MAX line on your machine.

4 Add a little water if needed to take it up to the MAX line.

5 Twist on the NUTRiBULLET blade and blend until smooth.

CHEF'S NOTE

For a creamy finish use almond milk instead of coconut water.

SERVES 1

SPICY TOMATO SMOOTHIE

255
calories

Ingredients

- 2 large tomatoes
- 1 red pepper
- ½ ripe avocado
- Dash of Tabasco/hot sauce
- Water

Method

1 Rinse the tomatoes & pepper. Core and roughly chop the pepper.

2 Peel and de-stone the avocado.

3 Add everything to the NUTRiBULLET tall cup. Make sure the ingredients do not go past the MAX line on your machine.

4 Add a little water if needed to take it up to the MAX line.

5 Twist on the NUTRiBULLET blade and blend until smooth.

CHEF'S NOTE

Tomatoes are an excellent source of vitamin C.

SERVES 1

HONEY & CHIA SEED SMOOTHIE

295 calories

Ingredients

- 75g/3oz strawberries
- 4 tbsp low-fat natural yoghurt
- 250ml/1 cup unsweetened almond milk
- 1 tbsp honey
- 2 tsp pumpkin seeds
- Water

Method

1 Rinse the strawberries and nip off any green tops.

2 Add them to the NUTRiBULLET tall cup along with the yoghurt, milk, honey & chia seeds. Make sure the ingredients do not go past the MAX line on your machine.

3 Add a little water if needed to take it up to the MAX line.

4 Twist on the NUTRiBULLET blade and blend until smooth. Pour into a glass and sprinkle with the pumpkin seeds.

CHEF'S NOTE

Try with any berries you have to hand.

THE Skinny NUTRiBULLET LEAN BODY YOGA PLAN

NUTRIBLASTS UNDER 400 CALORIES

SERVES 1

PAPAYA & BANANA SMOOTHIE

325 calories

Ingredients

- 50g/2oz spinach
- 1 banana
- 1 papaya fruit
- 150g/5oz fresh peeled pineapple
- 250ml/1 cup unsweetened almond milk
- Water

Method

1. Rinse the ingredients well.
2. Peel the banana and break into three pieces.
3. Scoop out the papaya flesh, discarding the seeds and rind.
4. Add the fruit, vegetables & milk to the NUTRiBULLET tall cup. Make sure the ingredients do not go past the MAX line on your machine.
5. Add water, again being careful not to exceed the MAX line.
6. Twist on the NUTRiBULLET blade and blend until smooth.

CHEF'S NOTE

Optional Nutriboost: Add 1 teaspoon of chia or flax seeds.

SERVES 1

AVOCADO SUPER GREEN SMOOTHIE

370 calories

Ingredients

- 50g/2oz spinach
- 1 apple
- ½ ripe avocado
- 250ml/1 cup semi skimmed milk
- Water

Method

1. Rinse the ingredients well.
2. Core the apple, leaving the skin on.
3. Scoop out the avocado flesh, discarding the stone and skin.
4. Add the fruit, vegetables & milk to the NUTRiBULLET tall cup. Make sure the ingredients do not go past the MAX line on your machine.
5. Add water, again being careful not to exceed the MAX line.
6. Twist on the NUTRiBULLET blade and blend until smooth.

CHEF'S NOTE

For a dairy free version use soya milk or unsweetened almond milk.

SERVES 1

BRIGHT HERB BLAST

340 calories

Ingredients

- 50g/2oz spinach
- 2 apples
- 1 tbsp lime juice
- 10 fresh basil leaves
- 250ml/1 cup unsweetened almond milk
- Water

Method

1. Rinse the ingredients well.
2. Core the apples, leaving the skin on.
3. Add the fruit, vegetables, lime juice, basil & milk to the NUTRiBULLET tall cup. Make sure the ingredients do not go past the MAX line on your machine.
4. Add water, again being careful not to exceed the MAX line.
5. Twist on the NUTRiBULLET blade and blend until smooth.

CHEF'S NOTE

Optional Nutriboost: Add 1 tablespoon of fresh almonds.

SERVES 1

GREEN GRAPE GOOD JUICE

340 calories

Ingredients

- 50g/2oz spinach
- 1 pear
- 1 apple
- 200g/7oz fresh seedless green grapes
- Water

Method

1 Rinse the ingredients well.

2 Core the pear and apple, leaving the skin on.

3 Remove any stalks from the grapes.

4 Add all the fruit & vegetables to the NUTRiBULLET tall cup. Make sure the ingredients do not go past the MAX line on your machine.

5 Add water, again being careful not to exceed the MAX line.

6 Twist on the NUTRiBULLET blade and blend until smooth.

CHEF'S NOTE

This is a really light fresh juice.

SERVES 1

GRAPEFRUIT & PINEAPPLE SWEET JUICE

335 calories

Ingredients

- 1 grapefruit
- 1 apple
- 200g/7oz fresh peeled pineapple
- 1 tsp honey
- Water

Method

1 Rinse the ingredients well.

2 Peel the grapefruit and divide into segments, don't worry about the pips.

3 Core the apple.

4 Add all the fruit & vegetables to the NUTRiBULLET tall cup. Make sure the ingredients do not go past the MAX line on your machine.

5 Add water, again being careful not to exceed the MAX line.

6 Twist on the NUTRiBULLET blade and blend until smooth.

CHEF'S NOTE

Optional Nutriboost: Add 1 teaspoon of sunflower seeds.

SERVES 1

PEACH CASHEW SMOOTHIE

370 calories

Ingredients

- 50g/2oz spinach
- 1 banana
- 1 peach
- 10 cashew nuts
- 250ml/1 cup unsweetened almond milk
- Water

Method

1. Rinse the ingredients well.
2. Peel the banana and break into three pieces.
3. De-stone the peach, leaving the skin on.
4. Add the fruit, vegetables, nuts & milk to the NUTRiBULLET tall cup. Make sure the ingredients do not go past the MAX line on your machine.
5. Add water, again being careful not to exceed the MAX line.
6. Twist on the NUTRiBULLET blade and blend until smooth.

CHEF'S NOTE

Cashew nuts are packed with vitamins, minerals and antioxidants.

SERVES 1

CARROT & KALE CLEANSER

305 calories

Ingredients

- 1 handful shredded lettuce
- 50g/2oz kale
- 1 apple
- 1 banana
- 150g/5oz carrots
- 1 tsp honey
- Water

Method

1 Rinse the ingredients well.

2 Remove any thick stalks from the kale.

3 Core the apple, leaving the skin on. Peel the banana and break into three pieces.

4 Nip the ends off the carrots.

5 Add the fruit, vegetables & honey to the NUTRiBULLET tall cup. Make sure the ingredients do not go past the MAX line on your machine.

6 Add water, again being careful not to exceed the MAX line.

7 Twist on the NUTRiBULLET blade and blend until smooth.

CHEF'S NOTE

Adjust the honey to suit your own taste.

SERVES 1

SPRING GOJI BERRY SMOOTHIE

325 calories

Ingredients

- 50g/2oz shredded spring greens
- 150g/5oz strawberries
- 1 banana
- 2 tbsp goji berries
- 250ml/1 cup unsweetened almond milk
- Water

Method

1 Rinse the ingredients well.

2 Cut the green tops off the strawberries.

3 Peel the banana and break into three pieces.

4 Add the fruit, vegetables, milk & goji berries to the NUTRiBULLET tall cup. Make sure the ingredients do not go past the MAX line on your machine.

5 Add water (if there's space), again being careful not to exceed the MAX line.

6 Twist on the NUTRiBULLET blade and blend until smooth.

CHEF'S NOTE

Use spinach if you can't get spring greens.

SERVES 1

CHIA & SOYA PINEAPPLE SMOOTHIE

375 calories

Ingredients

- 50g/2oz spinach
- 1 banana
- 100g/3½oz fresh peeled pineapple
- 250ml/1 cup soya milk
- 1 tsp chia seeds
- Water

Method

1 Rinse the ingredients well.

2 Peel the banana and break into three pieces.

3 Add the fruit, vegetables, seeds & milk to the NUTRiBULLET tall cup. Make sure the ingredients do not go past the MAX line on your machine.

4 Add water, again being careful not to exceed the MAX line.

5 Twist on the NUTRiBULLET blade and blend until smooth.

CHEF'S NOTE

You could also try this with almond milk or coconut water.

SERVES 1

WALNUT BLUEBERRY SMOOTHIE

348 calories

Ingredients

- 50g/2oz spinach
- 1 banana
- 100g/3½oz blueberries
- 250ml/1 cup unsweetened almond milk
- 6 walnut halves
- Water

Method

1 Rinse the ingredients well.

2 Peel the banana and break into three pieces.

3 Add the fruit, vegetables, milk & nuts to the NUTRiBULLET tall cup. Make sure the ingredients do not go past the MAX line on your machine.

4 Add water, again being careful not to exceed the MAX line.

5 Twist on the NUTRiBULLET blade and blend until smooth.

CHEF'S NOTE

Walnuts are a good source of vitamin E, folate, melatonin, omega-3 fats, and antioxidants.

SERVES 1

CHERRY GREEN SMOOTHIE

380 calories

Ingredients

- 50g/2oz spinach
- 150g/5oz pitted cherries
- 1 banana
- 250ml/1 cup unsweetened almond milk
- 1 tbsp coconut oil
- Water

Method

1. Rinse the ingredients well.
2. Remove any thick stalks from the spinach.
3. Peel the banana. Make sure you have removed all the stalks and stones from the cherries.
4. Add the spinach, fruit & almond milk to the NUTRiBULLET tall cup. Make sure the ingredients do not go past the MAX line on your machine.
5. Add a little water if needed to take it up to the MAX line.
6. Twist on the NUTRiBULLET blade and blend until smooth.

CHEF'S NOTE

Pitted frozen cherries are a great shortcut ingredient for making this smoothie.

SERVES 1

PINEAPPLE PROTEIN SHAKE

390 calories

Ingredients

- 1 banana
- 200g/7oz fresh peeled pineapple
- 1 tbsp almonds
- 1 scoop protein powder
- Water

Method

1 Rinse the ingredients well.

2 Peel the banana and break into three pieces.

3 Add the fruit, almonds & protein powder to the NUTRiBULLET tall cup. Make sure the ingredients do not go past the MAX line on your machine.

4 Add water, again being careful not to exceed the MAX line.

5 Twist on the NUTRiBULLET blade and blend until smooth.

CHEF'S NOTE

Optional Nutriboost: Add 1 tablespoon of goji berries.

SERVES 1

FRESH ALMOND & PEAR SMOOTHIE

320 calories

Ingredients

- 1 pear
- 1 banana
- 250ml/1 cup unsweetened almond milk
- 1 tbsp almonds
- Water

Method

1 Rinse the ingredients well.

2 Core the pear, leaving the skin on. Peel the banana and break into three pieces.

3 Add the fruit, milk & almonds to the NUTRiBULLET tall cup. Make sure the ingredients do not go past the MAX line on your machine.

4 Add water, again being careful not to exceed the MAX line.

5 Twist on the NUTRiBULLET blade and blend until smooth.

CHEF'S NOTE

Optional Nutriboost: Add 1 teaspoon of hemp seeds.

SERVES 1

OAT & CHIA SEED MORNING BLASTER

310 calories

Ingredients

- 1 banana
- 1 tsp chia seeds
- 2 tbsp rolled oats
- 250ml/1 cup soya milk
- 1 tsp honey
- Water

Method

1 Rinse the ingredients well.

2 Peel the banana and break into three pieces.

3 Add the banana, chia seeds, oats & milk to the NUTRiBULLET tall cup. Make sure the ingredients do not go past the MAX line on your machine.

4 Add water, again being careful not to exceed the MAX line.

5 Twist on the NUTRiBULLET blade and blend until smooth.

CHEF'S NOTE

Try a handful of blueberries if you want to add some extra sweetness.

SERVES 1

BEETROOT & ORANGE PROTEIN SMOOTHIE

375 calories

Ingredients

- 150g/5oz beetroot
- 1 banana
- 250ml/1 cup orange juice
- 2cm/1 inch peeled fresh ginger root
- 1 scoop protein powder
- Water

Method

1 Rinse the ingredients well.

2 Peel the beetroot & banana.

3 Add the beetroot, fruit, juice, ginger & protein powder to the NUTRiBULLET tall cup. Make sure the ingredients do not go past the MAX line on your machine.

4 Add a little water if needed to take it up to the MAX line.

5 Twist on the NUTRiBULLET blade and blend until smooth.

CHEF'S NOTE

Protein powder is a super smoothie ingredient when you need some muscle building goodness.

SERVES 1

GREEN GREEN SOYA MILK SMOOTHIE

360 calories

Ingredients

- 50g/2oz spinach
- 50g/2oz kale
- 1 apple
- 1 banana
- 250ml/1 cup soya milk
- 1 tsp honey
- Water

Method

1 Rinse the ingredients well.

2 Remove any thick stalks from the kale.

3 Core the apple, leaving the skin on. Peel the banana and break into three pieces.

4 Add all the fruit, vegetables, milk & honey to the NUTRiBULLET tall cup. Make sure the ingredients do not go past the MAX line on your machine.

5 Add water, again being careful not to exceed the MAX line.

6 Twist on the NUTRiBULLET blade and blend until smooth.

CHEF'S NOTE

Green smoothies can take a bit of getting used to but the natural sweetness of the honey, apple & banana will make them much easier to enjoy.

SERVES 1

KALE & COCONUT MILK SMOOTHIE

388 calories

Ingredients

- 50g/2oz kale
- 100g/3½oz carrots
- 1 apple
- 1 banana
- 250ml/1 cup low fat coconut milk
- 1 tsp honey
- Water

Method

1. Rinse the ingredients well.
2. Remove any thick stalks from the kale and nip the end off the carrots.
3. Core the apple, leaving the skin on. Peel the banana and break into three pieces.
4. Add the fruit, vegetables, milk & honey to the NUTRiBULLET tall cup. Making sure they do not go past the MAX line on your machine.
5. Add water, again being careful not to exceed the MAX line.
6. Twist on the NUTRiBULLET blade and blend until smooth.

CHEF'S NOTE

Kale is a powerful green super-food.

SERVES 1

BANANA & HEMP SEED SMOOTHIE

365 calories

Ingredients

- 1 banana
- 125g/4oz strawberries
- 250ml/1 cup unsweetened almond milk
- 2 tsp hemp seeds
- 1 scoop protein powder
- Water

Method

1 Peel the banana.

2 Rinse the strawberries and nip off any green tops.

3 Place the ingredients in the NUTRiBULLET tall cup making sure the ingredients do not go past the MAX line on your machine.

4 Top up with a little water if you like. Twist on the NUTRiBULLET blade and blend until smooth.

CHEF'S NOTE

Hemp seed is rich in omega 3 and omega 6.

SERVES 1

VANILLA & DATE COCONUT SMOOTHIE

365 calories

Ingredients

- 125g/4oz spinach
- 1 tsp vanilla extract
- 250ml/1 cup light coconut milk
- 5 pitted dates
- Water
- Ice cubes

Method

1 Rinse the spinach well and place in the NUTRiBULLET tall cup.

2 Add the coconut milk, vanilla, dates and a few ice cubes. Make sure the ingredients do not go past the MAX line on your machine.

3 Add water if needed to take it up to the MAX line.

4 Twist on the NUTRiBULLET blade and blend until smooth.

CHEF'S NOTE

Use dried sweet pitted dates.

SERVES 1

ALMOND BUTTER SPINACH SMOOTHIE

385 calories

Ingredients

- ½ ripe avocado
- 1 tbsp almond butter
- 2 tsp flax seeds
- 125g/4oz spinach
- 250ml/1 cup unsweetened almond milk
- Ice cubes

Method

1 Rinse the spinach and roughly chop. Peel and de-stone the avocado.

2 Add all the ingredients to the NUTRiBULLET tall cup. Make sure they do not go past the MAX line on your machine.

3 Twist on the NUTRiBULLET blade and blend until smooth.

CHEF'S NOTE

Almond butter is good source of vitamin E, copper & magnesium.

SERVES 1

HEMP & ALMOND MILK SMOOTHIE

320 calories

Ingredients

- 1 banana
- 2 tsp hemp seeds
- 250ml/1 cup unsweetened almond milk
- 1 tsp honey
- 1 tbsp almonds
- Water

Method

1 Rinse the ingredients well.

2 Peel the banana and break into three pieces.

3 Add the fruit, milk, honey, hemp seeds & almonds to the NUTRiBULLET tall cup. Make sure the ingredients do not go past the MAX line on your machine.

4 Add water, again being careful not to exceed the MAX line.

5 Twist on the NUTRiBULLET blade and blend until smooth.

CHEF'S NOTE

This delicious smoothie packs a double almond punch. Increase the honey if you wish.

YOGA Workouts

We recommend trying to find the time to practice yoga every day. A daily session will boost physical & mental wellbeing. The three workouts which have been developed in this book can be undertaken any time of the day depending on your schedule - although you will find the Morning & Tummy Toning Yoga most suited to the day time (or when you need to be refreshed) whilst the restful sleep yoga is best suited for the very the end of the day.

The first two workouts will take around 15 minutes to complete. The third is a 30 minute relaxation session. All you need to get started is a mat, a block and pillows for support. That said there is not need to run out and buy any equipment at all. You can do any of these routines comfortably on a rug or carpet and the yoga block can be substituted for a small strong shoe sized box.

Yoga should never be approached as a competitive sport. It is a personal journey. Always listen to your body and never push yourself too hard. Concentrating on breathing is an extremely important part of yoga practice and you will learnt to use the rhythm of your breathing to help you move through the poses. Always move into poses on a breath exhalation and make sure you move slowly and methodically. Try to relax your facial muscles and jaw whilst tensing the muscles you should be concentrating on.

Restful Sleep Workout Tips:

When you are undertaking this workout try to concentrate on nothing other than your own breathing. Try not to alter it but instead just feel it's natural rhythm and depth. Inevitably your mind will jump around from thought to thought - seemingly uncontrollably. Try not to become frustrated by this. Instead notice where your mind is and each time gently bring your thoughts back to your breathing. This is a skill in itself and it won't come right away. Emptying your mind is not as easy as it sounds, but have patience with yourself. If you try to anchor your thoughts around your breathing and repeat this routine regularly you will learn to calm your mind and move towards a stillness which will benefit your long term well being.

Morning YOGA

- Pose 1: **COW**
- Pose 2: **CAT**
- Pose 3: **COBRA**
- Pose 4: **EXTENSION**
- Pose 5: **ELBOW TO KNEE**
- Pose 6: **BIND**
- Pose 7: **LOW LUNGE**
- Pose 8: **LOW LUNGE STRETCH**
- Pose 9: **LIZARD POSE**
- Pose 10: **HALF SPLITS**
- Pose 11: **TWISTED MONKEY**
- Pose 12: **SIDE PLANK**
- Pose 13: **MOUNTAIN POSE**

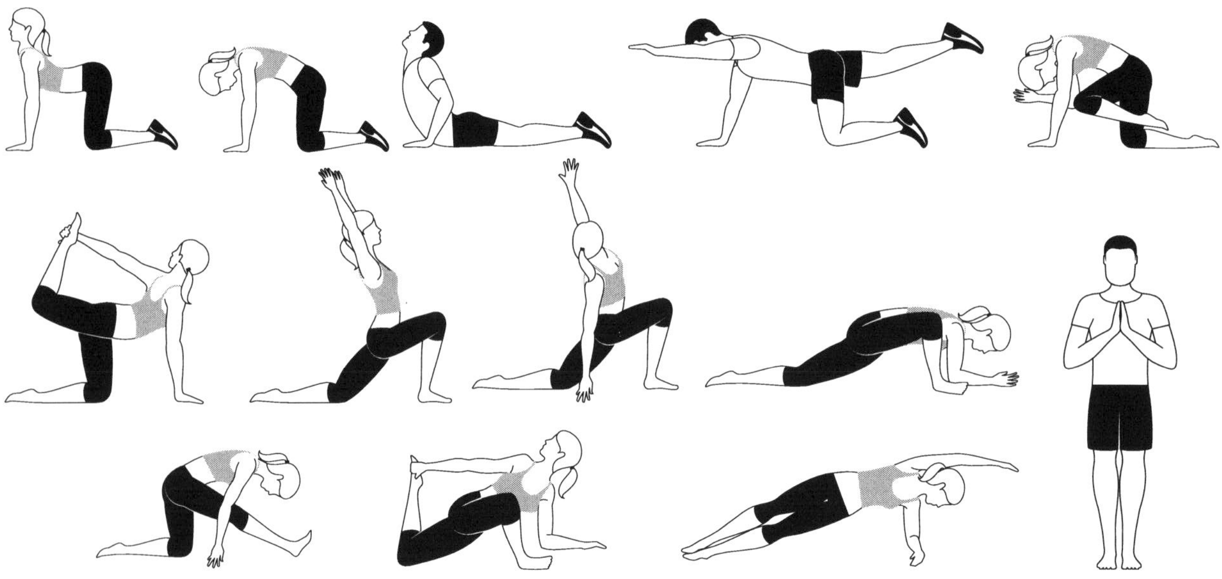

We have called this workout Morning Yoga as it is a wonderful routine to wake up with, but it can be used at any time throughout the day to refresh your mood and perk you up. It will take no more than 15 minutes and will prepare you for whatever lies ahead.

Cow

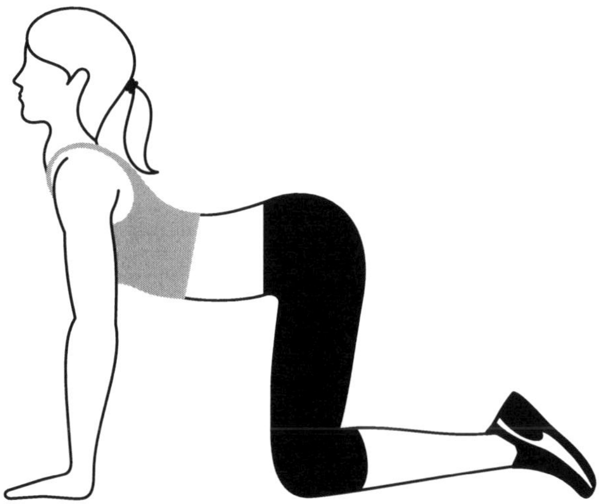

Come onto your hands and knees with hips placed over the knees. Shoulders positioned over the wrists. Your knees and hands should be shoulder distance apart, and the spine neutral. On exhalation gently lift your tail bone up to the sky, let your belly drop toward the mat and look up. Hold for a few moments before going into the next pose.

Cat

On a breath exhalation, lengthen your tail bone to the ground, draw the belly up to the spine and round the upper back like a cat. Concentrate on pressing your hands into the mat to open the shoulder blades. Let the head drop. Gently and slowly move through ten rounds of Cat/Cow, then return to a neutral spine.

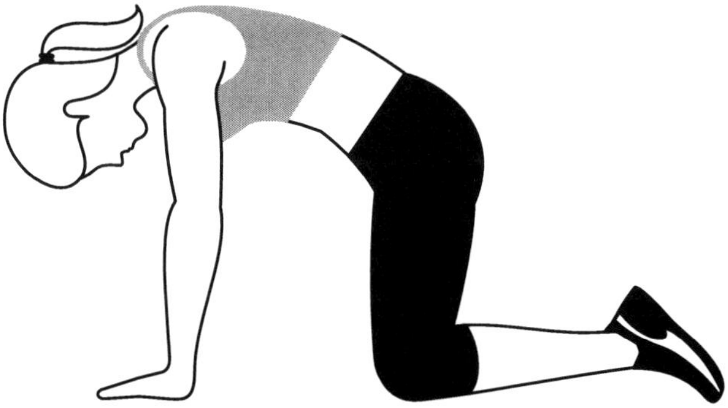

Cobra

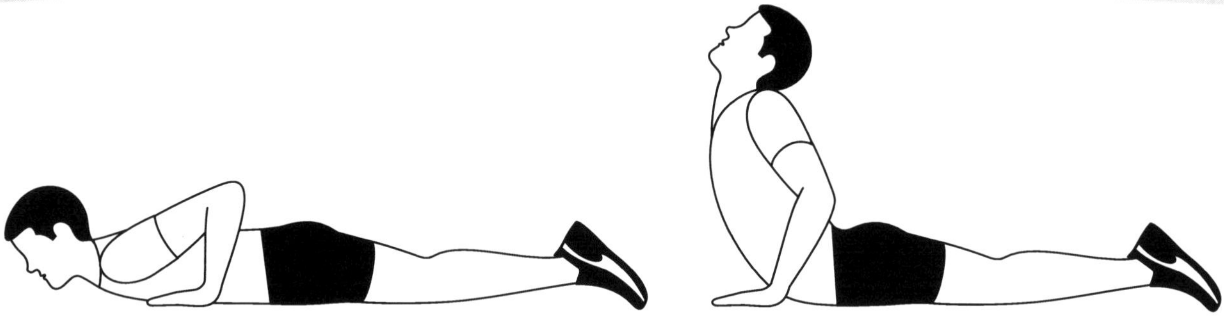

Lie face-down on mat. With elbows bent place the palms on each side of your body in line with the breastbone. Come onto fingertips and point elbows toward sky and out to sides. Press your pelvis, toes, and fingertips into the mat. On exhalation straighten the arms enough to fully lift the chest off the mat. Keep the spine long and tip the head back. Hold for 8 full deep breaths, engaging the thighs, before relaxing back onto the mat.

Extension

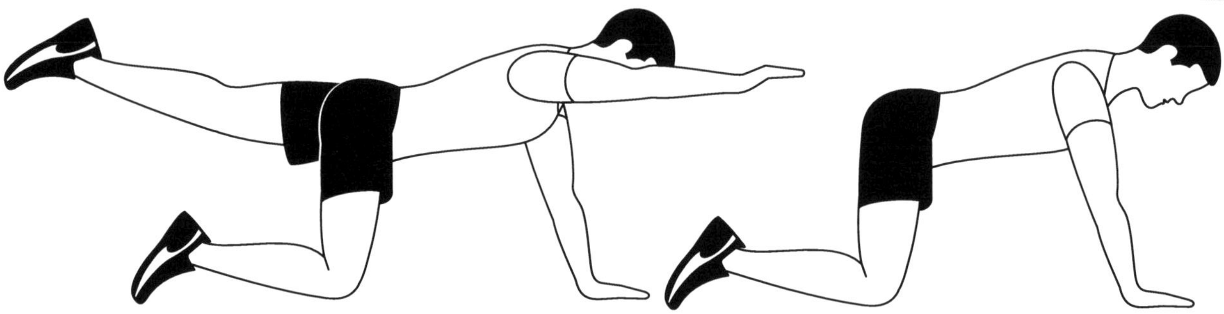

Move onto all fours. Lift your left leg and extend behind you whilst reaching your right arm forward. Lengthen your spine as you extend the arm and leg in opposite directions. Engage the core and maintain length in the back of the neck as you gaze down just in front of your hand on the mat. Hold for 5 long deep breaths. Reverse position and repeat.

Elbow To KNEE

From the extension pose move into the next pose by bringing your left elbow and your right knee in together to touch under the body. Do this on an exhalation and engage the core as you do so. Inhale to fully extend arm and leg into the extension pose and exhale to bring elbow and knee to touch. Repeat this in a careful measured way 5 times. Return to all fours ready for the next pose. Reverse position and repeat.

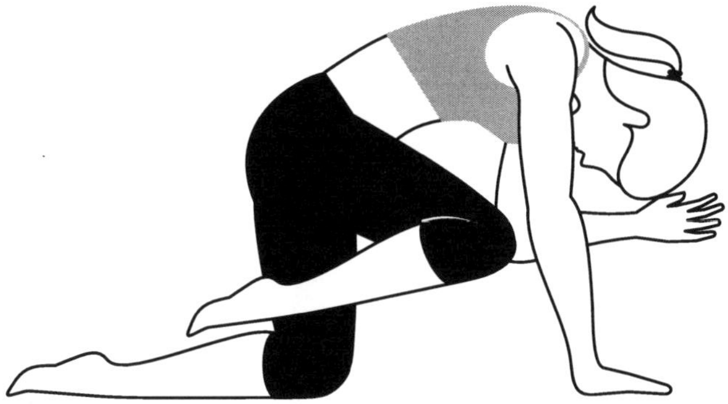

Bind

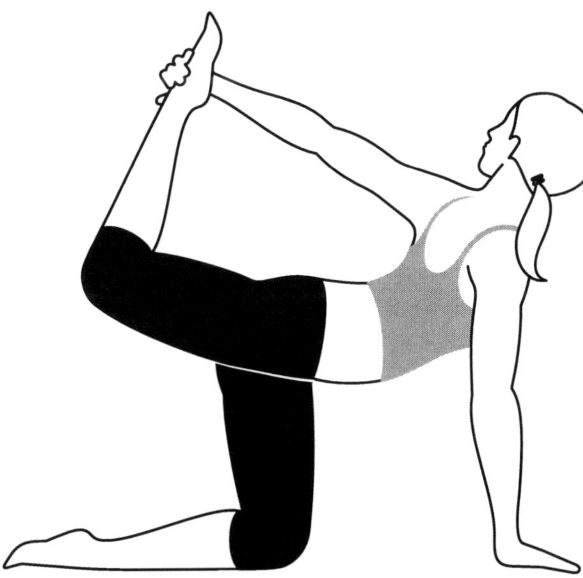

Reach left arm behind you and take hold of the right foot. Point the toes of this foot to the sky. Rolling the left shoulder toward the sky and draw the right shoulder back and down away from the right ear. Extend straight back from the hip. Hold for 5 slow deep breaths. Release from the pose. Lie on your back, hug knees to chest and gently rock side to side a few times to release the back. Reverse position and repeat.

Low LUNGE

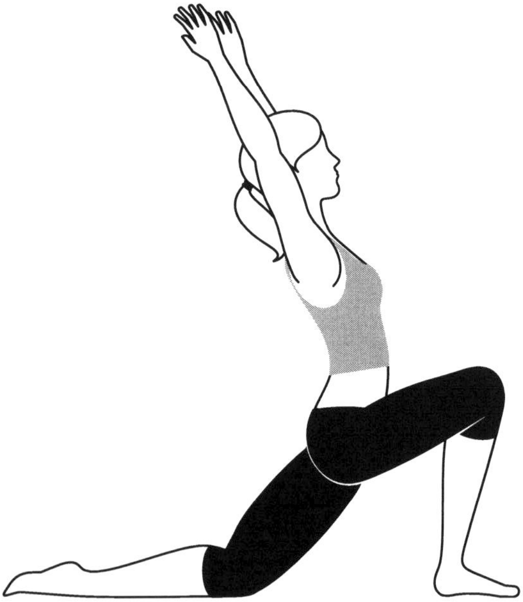

Stand straight on the mat with arms by sides. Step your right foot forward in between your hands, and on exhalation reach your arms up to the sky, keeping shoulders away from the ears. Push your right foot down and lower your hips towards the mat. Engage the core whilst avoiding puffing out the chest. Look forwards to the sky and hold the pose for 5 slow deep breaths. Reverse position and repeat.

Low Lunge STRETCH

From low lunge, reach your right fingertips down to the ground (you may wish to use a block). Exhale and reach up with the left fingertips for a full stretch. Concentrate on balance by pressing the right foot down into the mat. Look skywards but do not force your neck if this is uncomfortable. Keep the core engaged and the chest open. Feel the length of the stretch through your body and hold for 5 slow deep breaths. Reverse position and repeat.

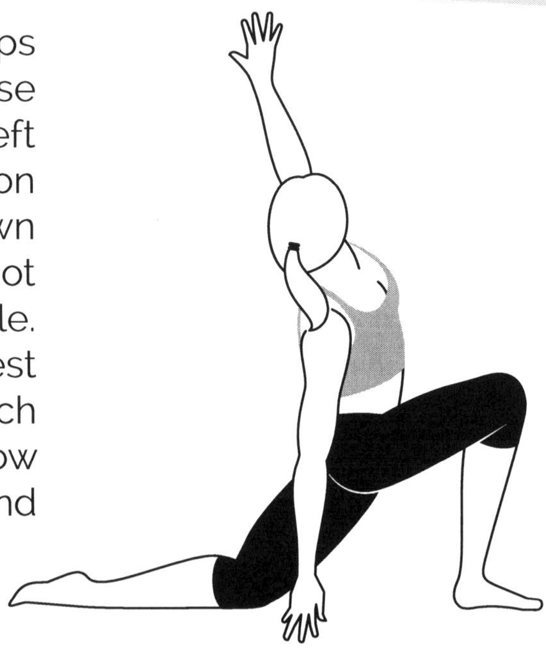

Lizard POSE

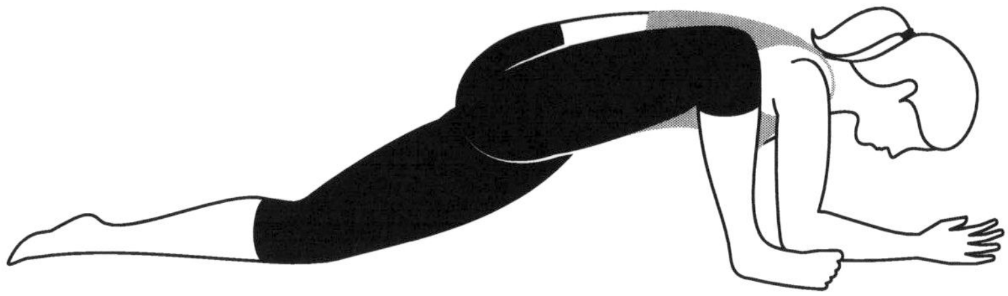

Move onto all fours on the mat. Bend the right knee and place the sole of the right foot into to the mat. On exhalation lower your body weight down to your forearms with palms facing each other. Move shoulders down away from the ears. Relax the right knee and allow it to rotate in the hip joint so that the knee falls to the right and the right foot is on its outer right edge. Do not force your knee down. Hold for 5 slow deep breaths before releasing from the pose. Reverse position and repeat.

Half SPLITS

Return to all fours. On exhalation slowly pull your hips back so that they are positioned over your left knee whilst straightening the right leg, Press your right heel into the mat, lengthen the right leg and flex the toes of the right foot back towards you. Keep the neck straight and look to the floor. Engage the core and hold for 5 slow deep breaths. Reverse position and repeat.

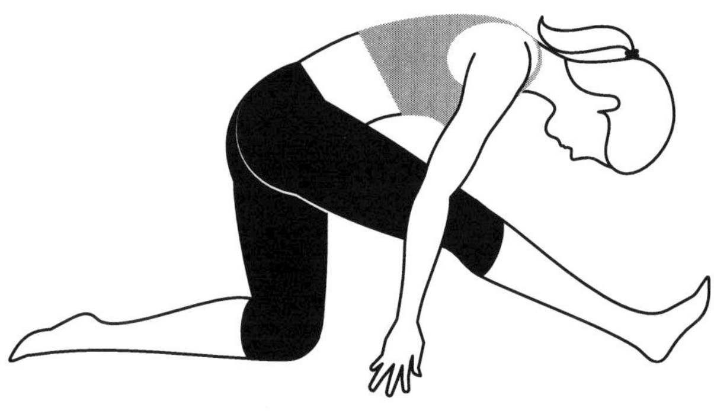

Twisted MONKEY

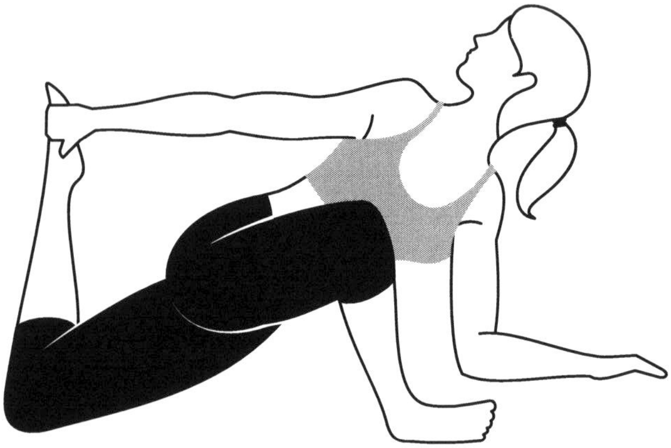

Return to all fours. On exhalation reach the right arm up and then back to take hold of your left foot. Roll the right shoulder back opening the chest. The left forearm should be flat on the mat with the palm extended. Allow the right knee to gently drop towards the floor as you come onto the outer edge of your right foot. Carefully lean the upper body back and hold for 5 slow deep breaths. Reverse position and repeat.

Side PLANK

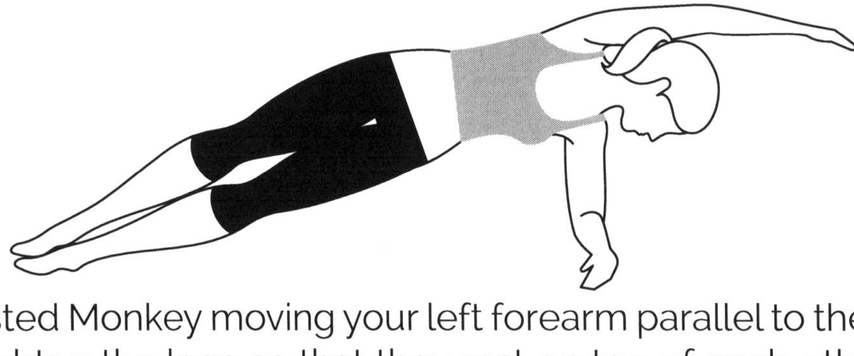

From Twisted Monkey moving your left forearm parallel to the top of the mat. Straighten the legs so that they rest on top of each other. Engage the core, extend the left arm over your head and lift the weight of your body to move into the side plank position. Feel the stretch through the side body and hold for 5 slow deep breaths. If you need stability split your legs so that both feet touch the floor. Reverse position and repeat.

Mountain POSE

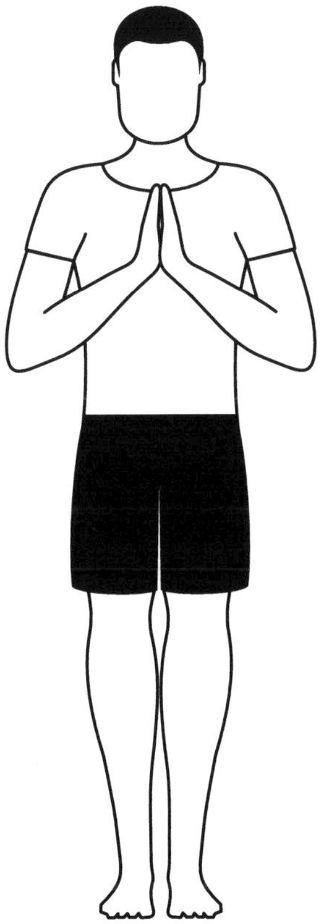

Finish the session with Mountain Pose by standing straight with legs and feet together, heels slightly apart, and arms at sides with palms facing forward. Keep your spine long, shoulders rolled back and away from the ears, spread the toes and press soles of the feet into mat. Engage thighs and lower belly, bring the gaze of the eyes towards the floor some distance ahead of you and lightly close the eyes. Slowly bring hands together at the centre of the chest and hold for 10 long deep breaths.

Tummy Toning YOGA

- Pose 1: **MOUNTAIN POSE**
- Pose 2: **STANDING LEAN**
- Pose 3: **COBRA**
- Pose 4: **MOUNTAIN CHAIR**
- Pose 5: **WARRIOR POSE**
- Pose 6: **CHEST OPENER**
- Pose 7: **DOWNWARD DOG**
- Pose 8: **PARTIAL PLANK**
- Pose 9: **PARTIAL SIDE PLANK**

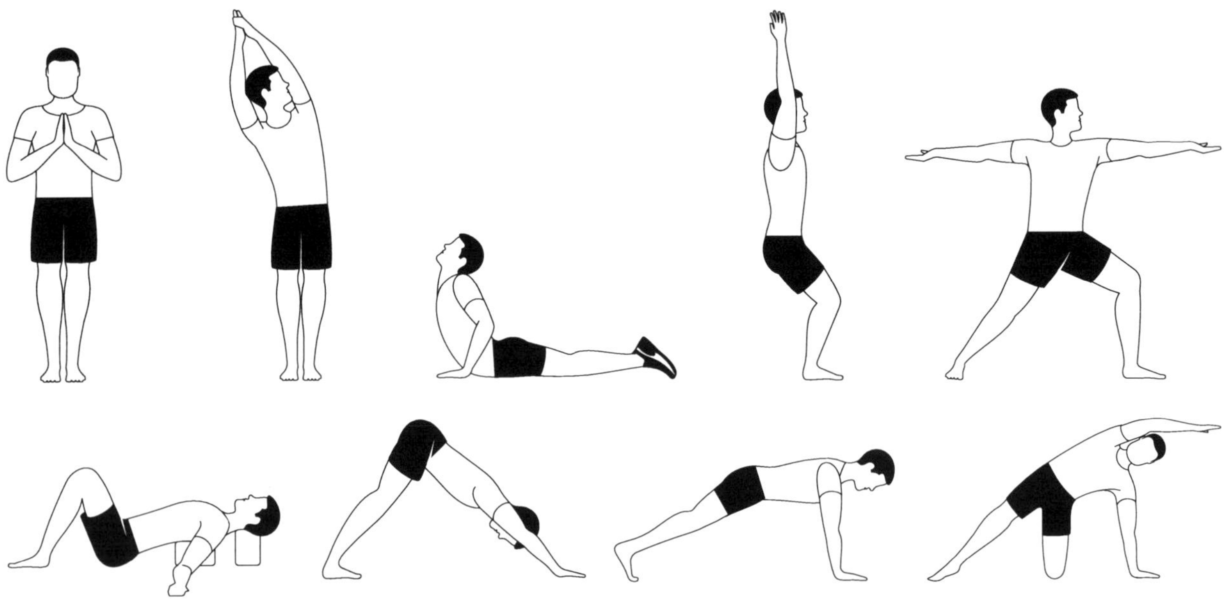

This routine is ideal for helping to tighten your core and it's also good for the thighs. Each of the poses will encourage you to use many of the core muscles we often forget about and should take no more than 30 minutes.

Mountain POSE

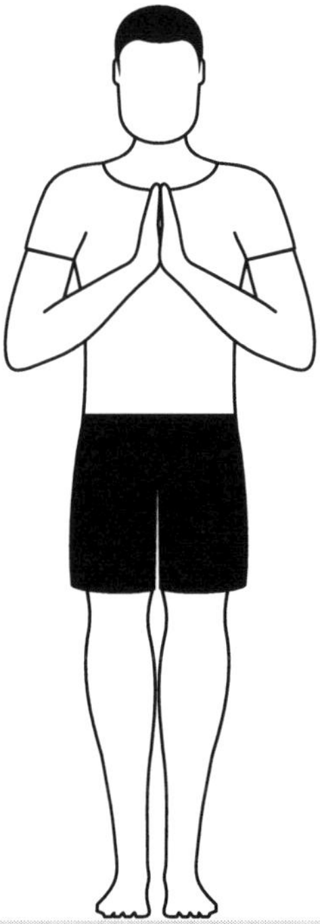

Begin the session with this iconic yoga pose by standing straight with legs and feet together, heels slightly apart, and arms at sides with palms facing forward. Keep your spine long, shoulders rolled back and away from the ears, spread the toes and press soles of the feet into mat. Engage thighs and core, bring the gaze of the eyes towards the floor some distance ahead of you and lightly close the eyes. Slowly bring hands together at the centre of the chest and hold for 10 long deep breaths.

Standing LEAN

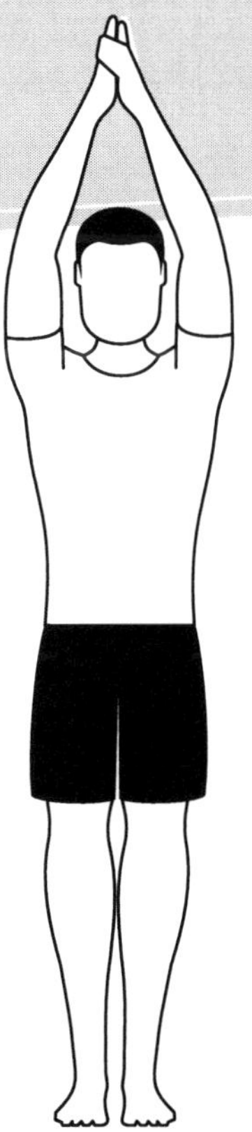

Begin by gently joining the palms above the head with the arms straight. Squeeze the inner arms in toward the ears but keep the shoulders down away from the ears. On your breath exhalation, press feet down, engage thighs and core, and stretch up and evenly over to right. Repeat the pose this time on the left side. Remember to engage the core and thighs each time and move on exhalation. Do this slowly on each side 4 times.

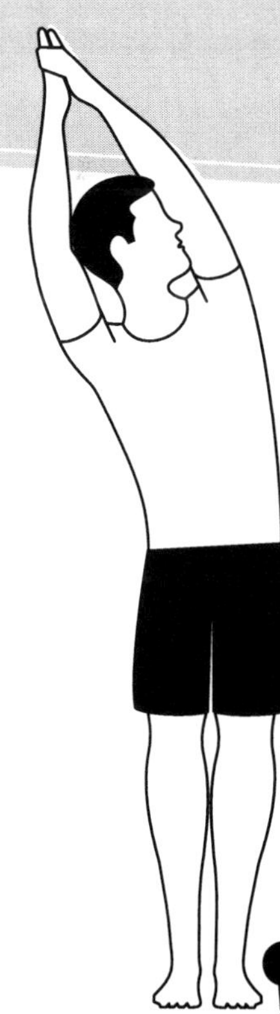

Cobra

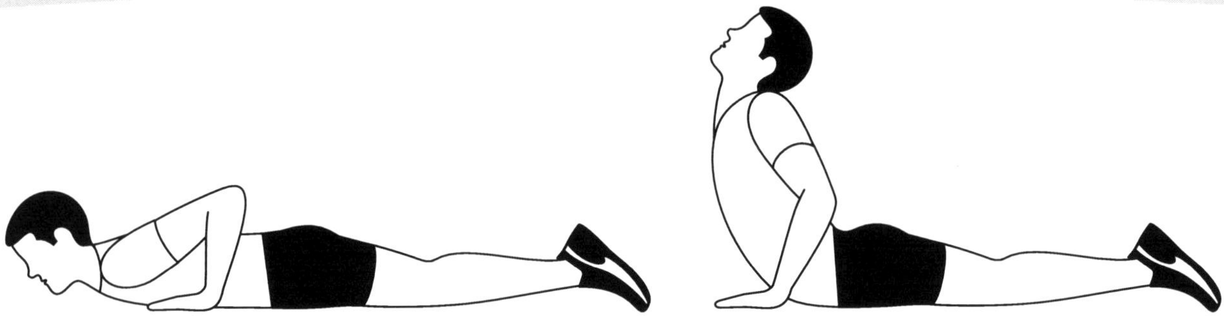

Lie face-down on mat. With elbows bent place the palms on each side of your body in line with the breastbone. Come onto fingertips and point elbows toward sky and out to sides. Press your pelvis, toes, and fingertips into the mat. On exhalation straighten the arms enough to fully lift the chest off the mat. Keep the spine long and tip the head back. Hold for 8 full deep breaths, engaging the core & thighs, before relaxing back onto the mat.

Mountain CHAIR

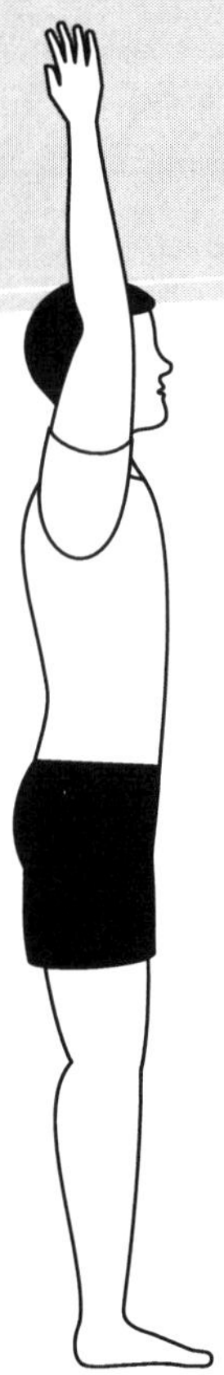

Stand straight with arms above the head and palms facing each other. On exhalation, sweep arms down and behind your body, bending knees and lowering hips. Inhale and reach arms overhead, biceps by ears with palms turned in toward each other, and sit into chair pose strongly engaging the core. On your next exhalation return to start. Repeat 10 times in a slow measured way.

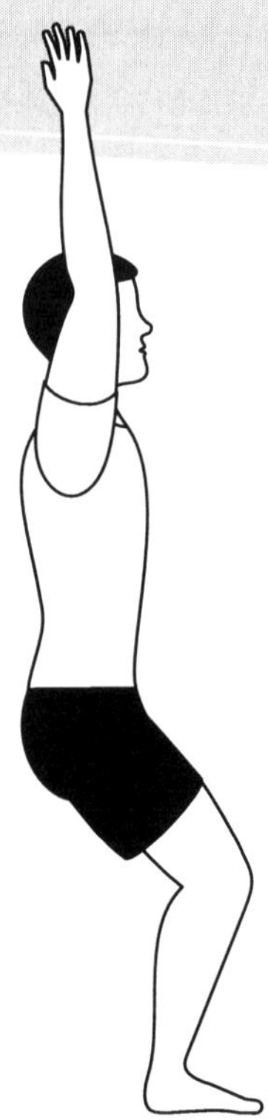

Warrior POSE

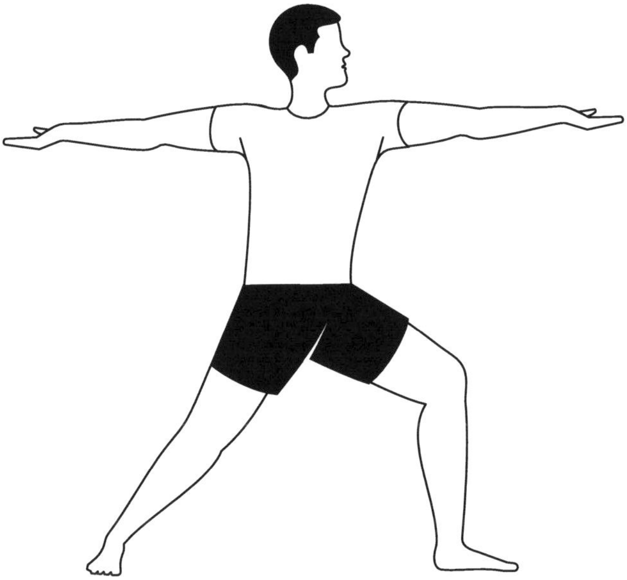

Extend the arms out at shoulder height and step your feet apart so they are positioned below the extended wrists. Have the outer edge of back foot parallel to back of mat and toes of front foot pointing forward. Engage the core and slowly bend front knee, lining it up over front ankle, and come into warrior pose with palms up.

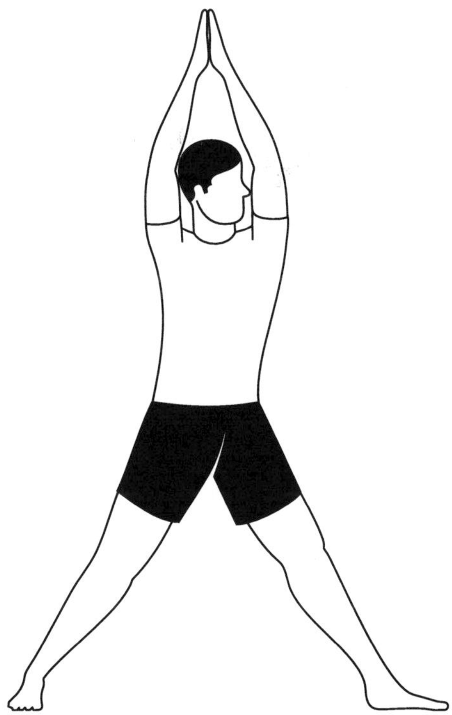

On exhalation, straighten your front leg and sweep the arms overhead, bringing palms together . On inhalation, return to warrior pose. Repeat 8 times. Switch legs and repeat.

Chest OPENER

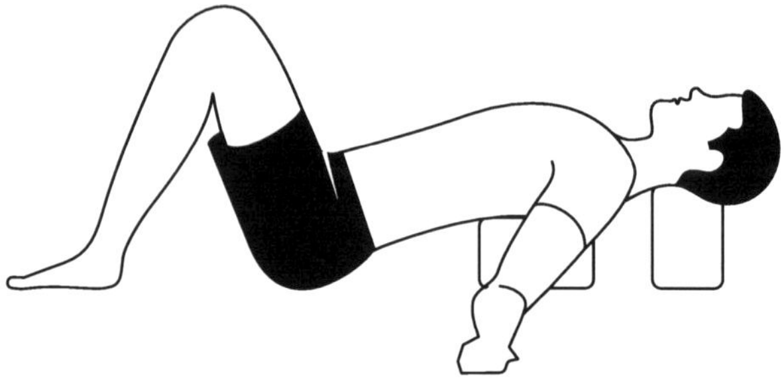

Lie face-up on mat with knees bent and feet positioned hip-width apart. Place a yoga block beneath your head and another lengthwise between shoulder blades. Bring arms out to sides and allow your chest to open. Engage your core strongly. Breathe through your stretch and stay in this pose for 2 minutes.

Downward DOG

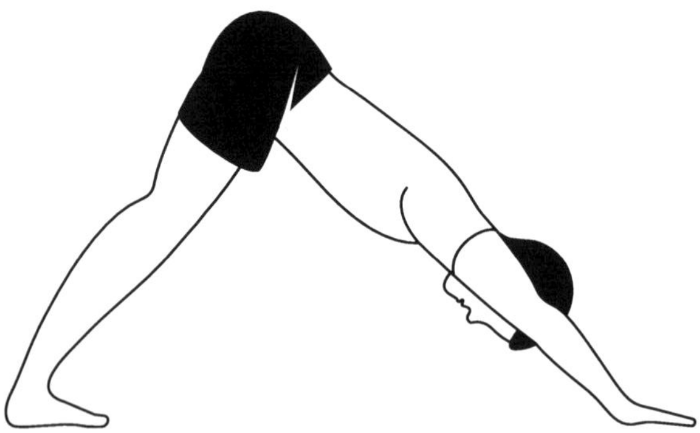

Start on all fours with knees and hands hip-width apart . Curl the feet to push toes into mat. On exhalation push down into hands and feet. Engage the core strongly and lift hips to sky keeping the back straight as if you are trying to push the mat away from yourself with your hands. Press down strongly through arms and balls of feet and lower heels onto the mat (don't worry if you have to bend your knees a little). Hold for 5 deep breaths keeping the core and thighs engaged throughout.

Partial PLANK

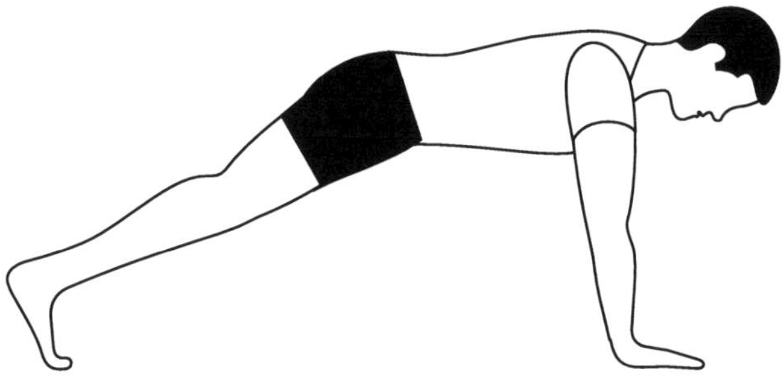

From Downward Dog, exhale and bring your body forward to come into the pose. Lengthen your spine and press heels towards the back of the room, engaging your core and thighs. Hold this position for a few moments then on exhalation, push down back into the downward dog pose. Keep the core and thighs engaged as you repeat this slowly 7 times.

Partial Side PLANK

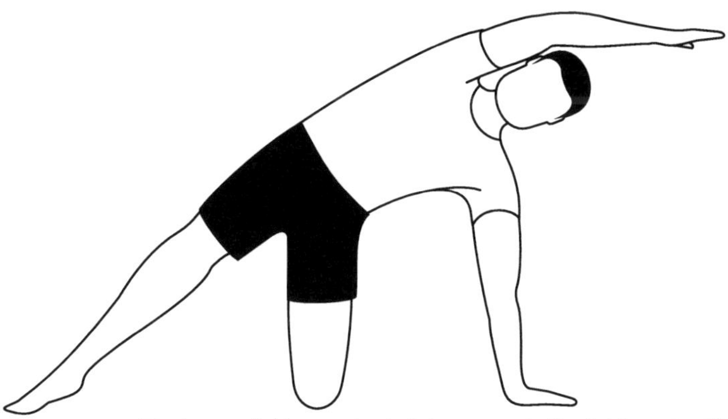

Move onto your knees. Extend the right leg whilst the left stays rooted to the floor. On exhalation turn your body to the right, shifting your weight onto left palm and right foot. Keep your spine and neck in line as you extend the right arm overhead, with palm facing down. Hold for 8 full deep breaths. Repeat on opposite side.

Restful Sleep YOGA

- Pose 1: **COW**
- Pose 2: **CAT**
- Pose 3: **BRIDGE POSE**
- Pose 4: **LEGS UP THE WALL**
- Pose 5: **SEATED FORWARD BEND**
- Pose 6: **WIDE LEG FORWARD BEND**
- Pose 7: **COBRA**
- Pose 8: **LEFT NOSTRIL BREATHING**

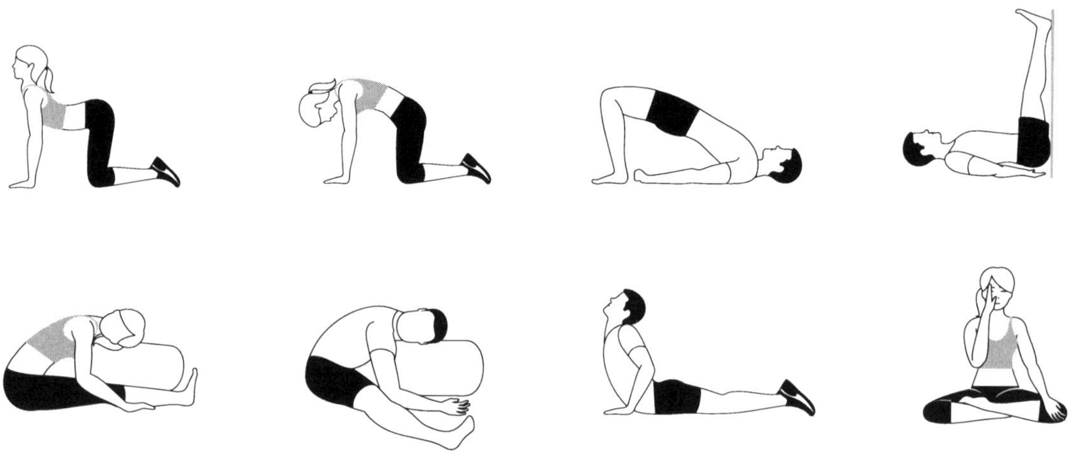

This gentle routine is ideal for preparing for bed, winding down in the evening or if you wish to meditate/rest throughout the day. You will need to have a mat and some pillows to hand and it should take no more than 30 minutes. Feel free to lengthen or shorten each of the poses to suit your own schedule.

Cow

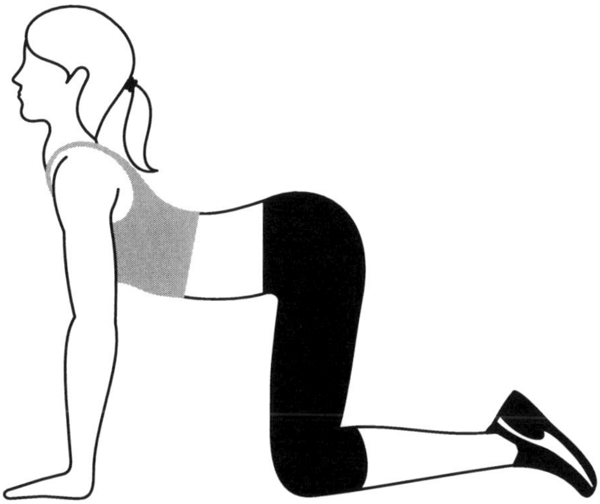

Come onto your hands and knees with hips placed over the knees. Shoulders positioned over the wrists. Your knees and hands should be shoulder distance apart, and the spine neutral. On exhalation gently lift your tail bone up to the sky, let your belly drop toward the mat and look up. Hold for a few moments before going into the next pose.

Cat

On a breath exhalation, lengthen your tail bone to the ground, draw the belly up to the spine and round the upper back like a cat. Concentrate on pressing your hands into the mat to open the shoulder blades. Let the head drop. Gently and slowly move through ten rounds of Cat/Cow, then return to a neutral spine.

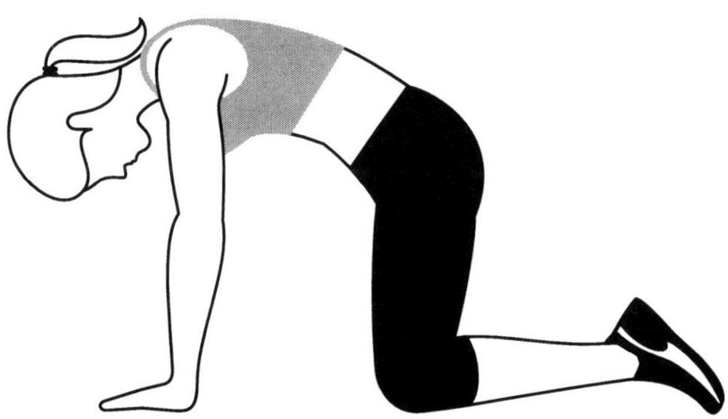

Bridge POSE

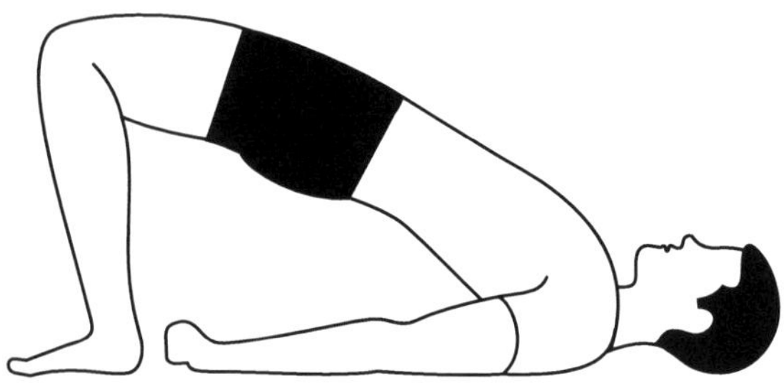

On your mat lie down with feet flat on the floor hip-width apart. Place your hands beside you with palms facing down. Engage your thighs and core and on exhalation lift your body up so that your back is flat and your knees are at a 45 degree angle whilst your arms remain flat on the floor. Settle into the pose and hold it for 2-3 minutes if you can.

Legs Up THE WALL

Position yourself on your mat side-on close up to wall. Roll onto your back with your legs up in the air. Twist yourself around 90 degrees so that your legs rest straight up against the wall. Shuffle your bottom up tight against the wall if you need to. Keep your arms straight by your side with the palms flat down. Remain in this pose for 5 minutes breathing deeply and slowly, concentrating on nothing other than movement and feeling of your breath.

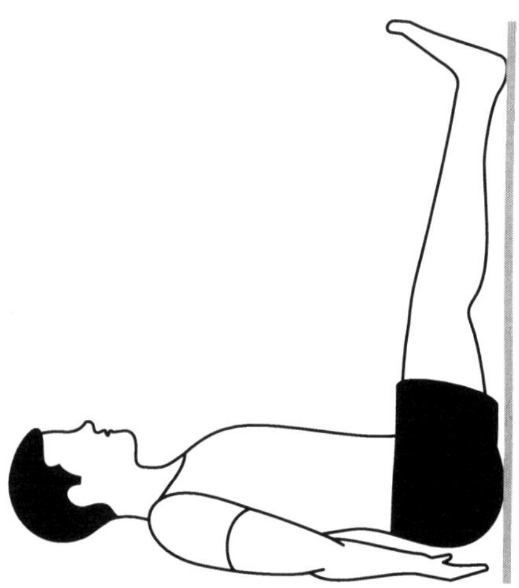

Seated Forward BEND

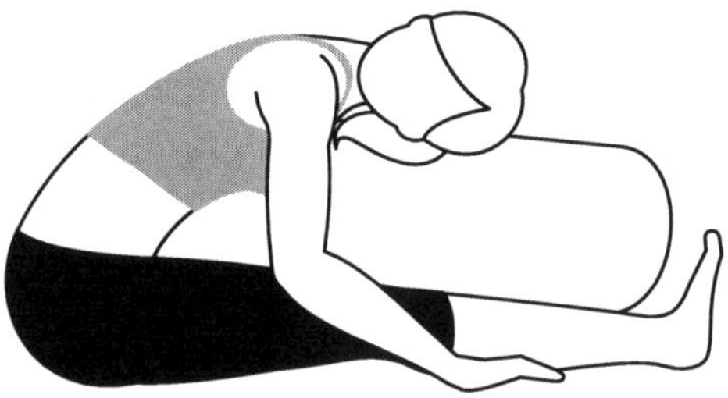

Sit on the mat with your legs straight out in front of you. Place pillow(s) on your thighs against your stomach (you may need to experiment with the height of the support). Put your arms above your head then reach forward as you bend your body onto the pillow and rest the side of your head onto the pillow support. Allow your arms to rest by your side and remain in this position for 5 minutes.

Wide Leg Forward BEND

This is a variation on the last pose. This time move your legs apart whilst you are in an upright sitting position. Place your cushion(s) onto the floor between your legs. Put your arms above your head then reach forward as you bend your body onto the pillow and rest the side of your head onto the pillow support – use the opposite side of your head from the last pose. Allow your arms to rest by your side and remain in this position for 5 minutes. If this feels uncomfortable it can be helpful to sit on a block or cushion to lift your pelvis or/and you may wish to bend your knees a little.

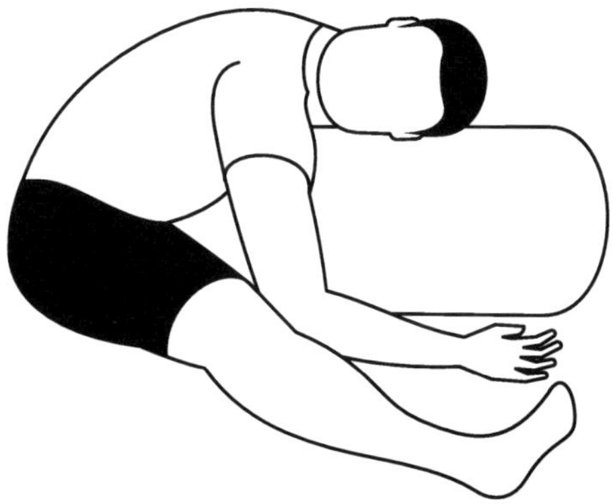

Cobra

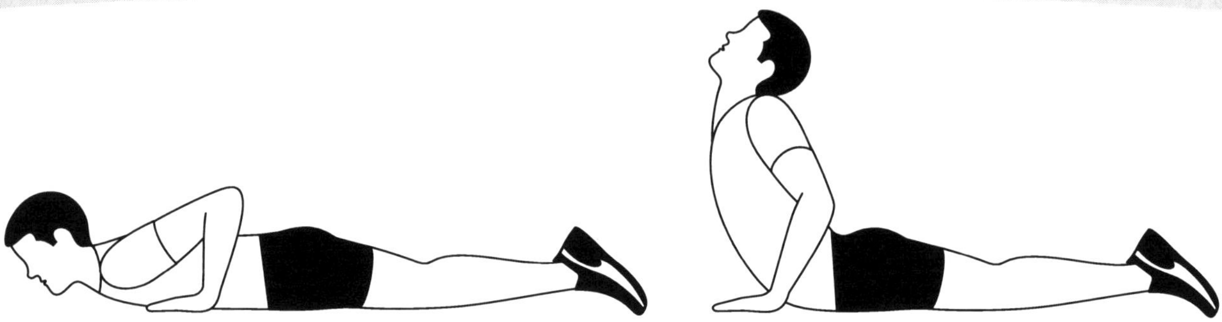

Lie face-down on mat. With elbows bent place palms a little away from each side of your body in line with the breastbone. Come onto fingertips and point elbows toward sky and out to sides Press pelvis, toes, and fingertips into floor. On exhalation straighten the arms enough to lift the chest off the mat. Keep the spine long and tip the head back. Hold for 8 full deep breaths before relaxing back onto the mat.

Left Nostril BREATHING

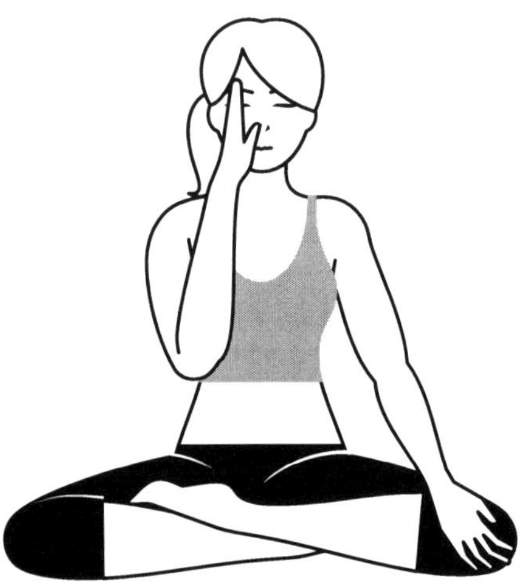

Sit in a comfortable cross- legged position. Keep your back straight with your shoulders low down away from your ears. Try to imagine a piece of string being pulled from above lifting the crown of your head up towards the sky. Cover your right nostril with your thumb or finger and begin breathing in and out through your left nostril. Breathe like this for at least 2 minutes.

This may seem strange but breathing through the left nostril has a calming effect on the nervous system and aids mediation and restful sleep.

Other COOKNATION TITLES

If you enjoyed **The *Skinny* NUTRiBULLET Lean Body *Yoga* Plan** you may also be interested in other *Skinny* **NUTRiBULLET** titles in the CookNation series.

Visit **www.bellmackenzie.com** to browse the full catalogue.

28329260R00055

Printed in Great Britain
by Amazon